The Doctor's Communication Handbook

PETER TATE

Examiner, Royal College of General Practitioners

Provided as an educational service by

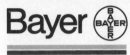

Radcliffe Medical Press
Oxford and New York

© 1994 Radcliffe Medical Press Ltd
18 Marcham Road, Abingdon, Oxon, OX14 1AA, UK

Radcliffe Medical Press, Inc.
141 Fifth Avenue, New York, NY 10010, USA

Reprinted 1995

British Library Cataloguing in Publication Data

A catalogue record for this book is available from the British Library.

ISBN 1 85775 011 X

Typeset by Tradespools Ltd, Frome, Somerset
Printed and bound in Great Britain by TJ Press, Padstow, Cornwall

Contents

Contents

Acknowledgements

This book would not have been written without Mark Mayall's insistence. I owe a great debt to all the other trainees who have stimulated me so much over the years. There is David Pendleton who first showed me the way and still points to the path. There are Peter Havelock and Theo Schofield who remain a constant source of inspiration, and also my great American friends, Professor David Smith and Professor Paul Arntson. I owe much to Peter Pritchard who has kept pushing me, and to Goran Aman who keeps taking me to Sweden to meet other stimulating colleagues. I should mention the legion of researchers and writers whose ideas I have shamelessly plagiarized without acknowledgement in order to keep the book easily readable. I owe a large debt to Roger Neighbour, Peter Campion, David Haslam, Richard Wakeford, and other members of the RCGP panel of examiners who never cease to inspire me with their constant enquiry and search for excellence, and most of all to John Foulkes, the friendly academic with the razor sharp mind, to whom this little tome is dedicated.

Foreword

The teaching and learning of communication in medicine has recently been the subject of a great deal of attention. While some commentators may see this emphasis as a fashion or bandwagon, others recognize that it signifies a real change in the way in which health care will be delivered in the future. There is a growing body of evidence that poor communication leads to poor outcomes for the patient. As for the process of the consultation, we know that more than half of patients' complaints and concerns are not elicited by doctors and that psychiatric and psychosocial problems are missed in up to 50 per cent of cases. Patients and doctors do not agree about the nature of the main presenting problem in about 50 per cent of encounters: is it therefore not suprising that most complaints about doctors by the public are about communication rather than clinical competence?

This book is written by an enthusiast who has been convinced of the importance of communication in improving health outcomes for the past 20 years. He has been involved in pioneering work in studying the consultation, he devised the consultation map first published in 1984, and has continued to develop his ideas within the panel of examiners for the MRCGP. I have worked with him for the past 10 years and it is a pleasure to introduce this handbook which is such an excellent synthesis of theory and practice. All of the relevant concepts are included and the reader is directed to the academic underpinnings of the approach through further reading. However, the detailed instructions on how to learn more about one's own communication skills are the meat of the book. But best of all, the voice of the author speaks through the pages; you will be enthused, amused, irritated, informed and stimulated to review your own behaviour. Every time a clinician begins this process, the health outcome for some patient somewhere is likely to be better.

Lesley Southgate
Professor of General Practice
The Medical Colleges of Saint Bartholomew's
and the Royal London Hospital
February 1994

Preface

This book is intended to be read by medical students and general practice trainees; and should offer some help to any doctor wishing to improve their communication with patients.

It is the result of 15 years' experience of working with doctors and helping myself and them to understand and improve their ability to talk to patients. The bulk of the message derives from ideas contained in *The Consultation. An approach to learning and teaching*, but much of the presentation is new and several new concepts have been included.

I hope the book will be used like a small manual and opened frequently for reference especially when reviewing one's own performance.

Peter Tate
March 1994

CHAPTER 1

Some early truths to remember

1   The patient is as frightened as you are.

2   The patient thinks it is more serious than you do.

3   Illness is frightening, but understanding what is going on helps. This applies to the patient and to you.

4   Taking a history is a method of controlling what the patient says.

> This book is a guide to help you talk with, understand and share with your patients. It will not teach you the traditional medical history taking model, but may help you to use that model more effectively.

Those first encounters with real people who have come to hospital or the outpatients department for help are very daunting. We all suffer the anxiety of being found wanting, of getting it wrong, of being harshly criticized by our teachers, or worst of all, just looking foolish. Perhaps the best way to start is to think ourselves into the role of patient. This is not too difficult; we have all been ill at some time and we all will be again. When people become ill they ask themselves several questions, such as What has happened? Why has it happened? Why to me? Why now?

What should I do about it? Should I go to the doctor? Is it serious? Can it be treated? Think of the last patient you saw. What questions do you think they had asked themselves? Imagine that patient was you. What would you be asking yourself?

Let us suppose that the last patient you saw was in a surgical outpatient department, and she was a woman of 35 presenting to the clinic with a nodular goitre. You have taken her history and discovered that she is married with no children, she first noticed the swelling in her neck some six months ago, went to her GP three months ago and has been waiting for the outpatient appointment since her second visit to the GP two and a half months ago. The GP has said in his letter that the thyroid function tests were borderline normal and that there is no family history of thyroid disease. In your detailed and schematic history taking you have not discovered any symptoms referable to the thyroid gland, but she does seem a little anxious. Examination confirms a moderately enlarged gland with multiple small nodules. Everything else is normal but she is a little trembly and perhaps sweating more than you would expect. Now step aside from your history and examination and ask yourself what might she be thinking and feeling? OK? Now do it again.

Let us go over some of her possible thoughts and feelings. Firstly, she is almost certainly frightened. Hospitals are terrifying places to most people. They are pain and death boxes with a funny smell. She is also afraid of the staff, especially the doctors, including you. Doctors are frightening for several reasons, not least their associations with the mysteries of life and death. They also tend to be dominant powerful figures who have control over one's immediate and even long-term future. She knows that many doctors do not say very much and what they do say can be difficult to understand. She also knows that doctors usually do not tell the whole truth.

She is also concerned about herself. She has a lumpy enlargement in her neck and to her it is cancer until proved otherwise, and she will take a lot of convincing because her aunt died of cancer in the gullet and she had lumps in her neck. She remembers that her aunt's doctor lied to her aunt, and that the treatment was horrible and ineffective. She has heard vaguely about the thyroid gland and knows from a friend that one of the treatments is radioactive. This concerns her because she desperately wants children, she knows time is passing her by and she fears that a dose of radioactivity may put paid to her chances forever. She is also afraid of an operation because she has never been into hospital and hates the idea of being put to sleep. She does not wish to lose control, and she also knows from friends, TV and everyday experiences that operations can go wrong and the neck seems a pretty dodgy place. She wishes her husband were with her, but worries that he does not want to talk about her neck or her coming to the hospital. She wonders if she is now ugly and unattractive. The bottom line is that she does not want to die.

This is only an imaginative guess at some of our patient's feelings, but how much of this did your history reveal do you think? Is it important to know?

You recite the findings of your history and examination to your chief. She listens and asks both you and your patient — let us call her Mrs Arthur — a few clarifying questions, and examines the thyroid gland herself. She excuses herself to Mrs Arthur and discusses the options with you while the patient listens.

> 'Multinodular goitre is a difficult clinical area and probably the best treatment is to do nothing if the patient can accept the clinical deformity. Some centres use thyroxine replacement but you only get regression in 10–20% of cases. The real worry for the patient is cancer, isn't it Mrs Arthur?' Mrs Arthur, a little startled, nods in agreement. 'Cancer is not really a problem. The Framingham study did not find any in a 15 year follow-up of this sort of goitre, but it remains a theoretical risk and if you give enough of any thyroid gland to a pathologist he will find some sort of cancer. The real problem we have here with Mrs Arthur is of possible toxicity and which would be the best treatment. The GP's thyroid function tests were borderline high and Mrs Arthur's clinical state is possibly a little suggestive of hyperactivity. We should repeat the tests and, if highish, give her treatment with radioactive iodine. If that is not successful the next step would be operation.' She smiles at Mrs Arthur and leaves the room saying 'The student will explain it all to you. Don't worry, you are in good hands.'

How do you think you would do? What do you think her feelings would be on the way home? What might she say to her husband? Would she come back for the I131 treatment? How helpful was your history? Mrs Arthur will appear again later. Keep her in mind.

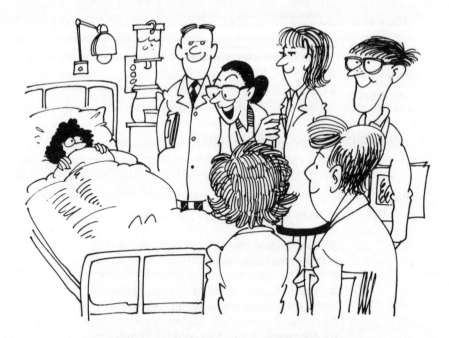

Think about yourself being unwell again. Imagine waking with a severe sore throat, lots of large neck glands and feeling pretty ropey. Would you go to your GP? If not, what else might make you go? What questions do you ask yourself?

Let us go through some of your possible questions and answers:

1 What has happened? It's probably just a virus, Max had it last week.

2 Why has it happened? I've been working late, a bit overtired, resistance is a bit low.

3 Why to me? Rotten luck, but I always get these things. Max sneezed over me.

4 What should I do about it? Dose myself up with soluble aspirin and it should just go.

5 Is it serious? No, it will be gone in a few days.

But what happens if the exams are two weeks away or there is a hockey trip to Lanzarote next week?

1   What has happened? Maybe it's a streptococcus.

2   What should I do about it? I'd better see the GP for some penicillin.

3   Is it serious? Yes, if I fail the exam or I can't make it to Lanzarote.

Or if your partner has glandular fever?

1   What has happened? Oh God, it's glandular fever.

2   Why has it happened? Too much kissing.

3   Why to me? I had it coming to me, life has been too good recently.

4   What should I do about it? I had better see the Doc to do a monospot to confirm it.

5   It is serious? Yes, this could put me out for the rest of the year. I've also read it can cause Hodgkin's disease. Oh my God!

These questions and answers can be translated into a trinity of *ideas, concerns* and *expectations*. To continue with the same example of the sore throat and glands scenario, think of what ideas might be going through your head that first morning ...

'I feel awful. Really really bad. Too bad for a cold. It must be 'flu at the very least. I bet I got it from Max, he was coughing and sneezing all over me last week. It might be streptococcal so a trip to the GP for some penicillin might help. I wonder if there's any on the ward I can have? I'll have to get some soluble aspirin' ... etc.

What concerns might be going through your brain?

'Help, I hope and pray it's not glandular fever. if it is, that's the exams down the tubes, and that can lead to Hodgkin's can't it? What if it's worse? I mean acute leukaemia can start like this. I've been worrying about my immune system for some time. I haven't caught AIDS in casualty, have I? Don't be silly, but it could turn into quinsy like that poor bloke on the ENT ward last week. His tonsils were so big he couldn't breathe. If I don't get this fixed pretty quickly, next week's trip to Lanzarote with the hockey team is finito'...etc.

What about your expectations?

'If I do nothing it'll probably go away. If I dose myself up, but penicillin is a good idea because it might speed things up, especially with the hockey trip coming up. I expect the old GP will just tell me it's a virus and I'll have to lay it on a bit thick to get the penicillin. He might do a blood test for glandular fever. Shall I tell him I'm a bit worried about AIDS? No, he'll think I'm silly. I expect he'll tell me off for smoking too'...etc.

Now think about Mrs Arthur again, and think about what sort of things were going through her mind before she went to her GP for the first time. What she did not do was to go to him with a nodular goitre. She went because she had ideas about the lumpy swelling in her neck, she had several concerns and a few hazy expectations.

Nobody goes to a doctor with just a symptom, they go with *ideas* about the symptom, with *concerns* about the symptom and with *expectations* related to the symptom.

CHAPTER 2

How doctors talk to patients and why

1 Asking questions only gives you answers.

2 Whether the communication between doctor and patient is 'good' or 'bad' is not as important as whether it is more or less effective.

For more than 3000 years, most doctoring can be described in ethical jargon as 'beneficient paternalism'. The medical profession has adopted a parental role in most encounters with patients. Doctors have acted on behalf of, and for the good of, their patients. They have also wielded power over them. This role, taken for granted by our society, produces recognizable patterns of behaviour which are disease oriented and self-protectively authoritarian.

There has been a great deal of research into doctors' behaviours and the reading list at the end of the book (*see* page 105) will help you to explore this area in more detail, should you wish to do so.

Agendas

One way of thinking about the ways in which doctors communicate is to think about agendas for both doctor and patient. Figure 2.1 demonstrates diagrammatically the possible spectrum of behaviours doctors may display when communicating with patients. The right hand column shows the doctor's agenda with only the presenting complaint coming from the patient. As the doctor's style of consulting becomes more patient-centred and moves to the left, more of the patient's agenda is taken on board until, in the left hand column, almost all the communication relates to the patient's agenda. The majority of doctors, whether in hospital or general practice, tend towards the right hand end of the model in their consulting style. This is not surprising as it is the way we are taught. The whole act of *taking* a history is doctor-centred, and not necessarily bad. Clinical thoroughness and good pattern recognition are hallmarks of this style practised well. As an example of doctor-centred behaviour, imagine Mrs Arthur's first out-patient appointment. It could go something like this.

> Doctor: 'Good morning Mrs Arthur. Your GP says you seem to have a problem with your thyroid gland. Tell me, have you lost weight?'
> Mrs Arthur: 'No.'
> 'Any hot flushes?'
> 'No.'
> 'Feeling tired or slowed up?'
> 'Er, well maybe a little Doctor.'
> 'Bowels OK, not constipated are you?'
> 'Not really Doctor. I was wondering . . .'
> 'I think I should examine you now. Would you take your blouse off . . .'

Mrs Arthur's agenda has not figured in the conversation so far; only the doctor's agenda has been addressed. Here is an example of a more patient-centred style, using the same scenario.

> Doctor: 'Good morning Mrs Arthur. Your GP says you have a problem with your thyroid gland. Would you tell me about it?'
> Mrs Arthur: 'Oh, er well yes. I first noticed the swelling a few months ago, but I didn't do anything about it for a while.'
> 'Why not?'
> 'Oh, you know, hoped it would go away while fearing the worst.'
> 'The worst?'
> 'Cancer, what else?'
> 'That's a frightening thought. Do you still think

it may be cancer?'
'Well yes, but I am hoping you will be able to
tell me Doctor.'

In this example, the patient's agenda figures highly to start with, and the doctor has not yet started on his agenda.

The totally patient-centred doctor is probably a dangerous creature. Patients do after all come for medical advice and considered professional opinions. They do not expect the doctor to let them do all the talking, planning and managing.

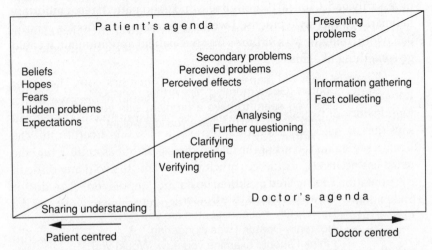

Figure 2.1: A power shift model of styles of consultation.

However, the first chapter may have started you thinking about how, in most consultations, the doctor should take on board some of the patient's belief systems. An ideal doctor lies in the middle, changing their behaviour to adapt to the needs of the patient and the situation. The problem is — shown by experience and research work — that doctors do not change. Audiotaping and videotaping of multiple consultations by the same doctor, show a remarkable consistency of style. A simple analogy likens us to the traditional Englishman abroad. We don't act differently, we just talk more loudly or more slowly. So doctors say and do things in much the same way with an anxious 16-year-old coming for a termination as a 50-year-old woman with menorrhagia or 80-year-old woman with vulval carcinoma. We do not adapt to meet the needs of the patient. You could say that this does not matter as long as we have an effective set of behaviours which will cope with most patients. However, Chapter 3 will demonstrate that different patients need different types of communication. We need to be flexible and it appears that most of us are not.

The most basic communication need is to discover why the patient has come to see you. This may seem obvious, but research suggests that doctors are not very good at this. In many consultations, doctors and patients do not appear to be talking about the same thing, ie they are dysfunctional. In dysfunctional consultations, the different agendas are not being met.

Doctors are good at diagnosis (ie in the medical sense why a patient has come to see you). We discover the nature and history of the problem and the likely cause, but we tend not to search out the patient's beliefs and expectations. These are the real reasons that the patient has come to see us. Not discovering them can lead to a mismatch of agendas. For example:

A gloomy 64-year-old man comes to his GP for a sick note. The doctor knows him to be a somewhat aggressive, paranoid depressive with a long history of repeated admissions to a mental hospital. The patient says that he has been in hospital recently and wants a certificate. The doctor, seeing no record of the latest admission, but assuming that the usual has occurred, acquiesces quickly. He wants to avoid any difficult confrontation and writes a certificate stating 'depression'. The doctor and patient briefly discuss convalescence and returning to work and the patient leaves.

What is wrong with this scenario? Almost everything! The whole consultation was based on a false premise. The patient had, in fact, been admitted to hospital with a myocardial infarction. The doctor's original assumption was false and nothing in the ensuing communication put this right. The doctor had failed to discover why his patient was there and the patient did not realize this.

Dysfunctional consultations are common in general practice and major misunderstandings can happen in hospitals. Consider Mrs Arthur again. Assume that the doctor has examined her and completed the history in a series of staccato questions. Mrs Arthur has, therefore, contributed none of her own thoughts and feelings. The time for explanation and management has come.

> Doctor: 'Well Mrs Arthur, there is nothing to worry about. You have multinodular goitre; however, this is a benign condition. There are a couple more tests we need to do to be on the safe side. I will arrange for a special scan and a

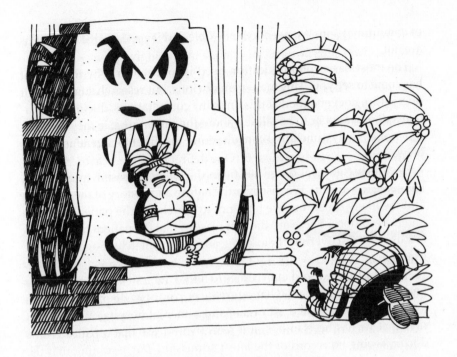

biopsy of that biggish lump. Is that OK?'
Mrs Arthur: 'So, you are sure it is not serious
Doctor?'
'Oh yes. Speak to the nurse about arrange-
ments for the tests and I will see you in a
month. Goodbye.'
'Well goodbye doctor, er thank you.'

This is a deficient communication. The patient has not had her agenda addressed. Consider her ideas from Chapter 1 (*see* page 2), and she has not been reassured about the future. She is not sure about the meaning of the words 'multinodular', 'goitre', 'benign', 'special scan' or 'biopsy', and she will go home frustrated and afraid. The doctor, in turn, has focused his attention on the thyroid gland to the exclusion of everything else. He knows little about Mrs Arthur and nothing of her specific fears or reasons for consulting.

Power

Look at Figure 2.1 again and think about power. This diagram is a power shift model; the doctor is much more in control on the right hand side, and his power slips away as the agenda increasingly becomes that of the patient. This is not to say that the totally patient-centred doctor does not have power. They simply have less control and are less authoritarian. It is worth stopping here to consider the nature of doctor power.

Patients expect and often want powerful doctors; that is a doctor who has reassuring authority, who is apparently capable and whose pronouncements can reduce anxiety. One definition of medical or 'Aesculapean' authority divides it into three parts: sapiental, moral and charismatic.

Sapiental authority

This can be defined as the right to be heard based on knowledge or expertise, and means that doctors must know or appear to know more about medicine than their patients. This can only be one part of the doctor's authority, however, as a biochemist may know more about a particular branch of medicine, but it is to a physician that a patient turns when in need.

Moral authority

This is derived from the Hippocratic credo in which society expects doctors to have a considerable degree of control over patients and to direct them for their own good. In addition, societies generally revere doctors, meaning that their behaviour is seen as socially right as well as individually good. This is a powerful combination.

Charismatic authority

This is the most difficult of the three concepts and is similar to the anthropological definition of magic. It stems from the original unity between medicine and religion. In Western culture it is related to the possibility of death and the magnitude of the issues with which the doctor deals. This is one reason for the priestly role adopted by some doctors, as it implies the desire to see the practice of medicine as something of a mystery, a desire to supplement sapiental and moral authority with an ineffable factor which might just hold out hope against the odds. Many doctors go out of their way to cultivate this. They develop a priestly mien, use complicated and obscure rituals, and act more like bishops than physicians.

These three forms of authority are present in all doctors, although some try to develop particular sapiental, moral and charismatic elements in their behaviour with patients and others. Think about some of the powerful doctors you have met and the nature of their power.

Here is an example. A partially patient-centred doctor in Figure 2.1 has the same moral authority as her doctor-centred colleague, but she may reduce some of her sapiental authority by sharing more information with her patients. Controlling information increases the doctor's power. Many doctors are uneasy with knowledgeable, inquisitive patients; such patients lessen the doctor's control. The partially patient-centred doctor will also be more likely to demystify the nature of medical diagnosis and treatment, reducing her charismatic authority and thus her power still further.

Many doctors, and perhaps especially when training, are afraid of losing control, of exposing too much of their patient's pain and fear, in case they open an emotional Pandora's box and become overwhelmed by what comes out of it. They use their power over the patient to keep the box shut and emotions at a non-threatening level. This style of behaviour then becomes fixed and can persist throughout their career. Do not let this happen to you. You will lose much more than you will gain.

Doctors can increase their charismatic power, should they wish, in many ways. The trappings of power are the most obvious. White coats, impressive and mysterious gadgetry, attached (subservient) staff, large desks with the big chair firmly behind it, grandiose looking certificates on the wall, computers with unintelligible displays or facing away from the patient, etc. Communication by cryptic oracle, like pronouncements shrouded in technical terminology and wrapped up with dire warnings on non-compliance, help to complete the effect. Powerful rituals such as examining and prescribing are more charismatic in the absence of adequate explanations.

The problem with this contrived exercise of medical authority is that overwhelming evidence suggests that it is not very effective. It quite obviously does not increase patient understanding because that is not what is motivating the doctor. The often quoted reason for this style of communication is that it will make patients do what is good for them. However, the sad fact seems to be that more than often they do not. The literature on compliance with medical advice reflects rather badly on doctors.

The *rule of thirds* describes this. It is easy to remember and is well authenticated: One third of patients take medical advice and act in accordance with it, to an extent whereby the advice is effective; One third of patients take heed of some of the advice, but not enough for it to be effective; One third just do not bother with the advice.

Think about this long and hard. You want to be the finest doctor in the land — to be able to recognize a yellow nail syndrome at 20 feet, to restore ailing patients to full vigour with your hard earned expertise — but two thirds of your patients do not follow your advice. How useful are you as a doctor? How can you make sure that this fate will not befall you? Do you have to be in absolute control? Read on.

CHAPTER 3

Different types of patients

The same words are often interpreted differently by different people.

The health belief model

This is the most researched and validated description of patients' beliefs about health and related matters, and has five main elements.

1   People's interest in their health and the degree to which they are motivated to change it varies enormously. (*Health motivation.*)

2   When considering specific health problems, people think very differently about how likely they are to be affected. For example, people who think that they are at high risk of developing lung cancer are more likely to follow advice about giving up smoking than those who do not think they are at risk. (*Perceived vulnerability.*)

   If a patient already has a health problem, then the perceived vulnerability relates to the degree to which they believe in the diagnosis and its possible consequences. For example, a patient is diagnosed as having irritable bowel syndrome and it is suggested that tension may be contributing to the condition. However, if the patient is convinced that pelvic inflammatory disease is the cause, they may fail to comply with subsequent management. This disbelief in what they are told may not be explicit and needs to be searched for.

3   Patients vary in how dire they believe the consequences of contracting a particular illness would be and what would happen if it were left untreated. (*Perceived seriousness.*) Heart disease or lung cancer can be seen as too far in the future to concern a teenage girl starting to smoke through peer pressure. Her attitude may be 'and anyway by the time I get to 40 they'll have a cure for it, won't they?'.

On the other hand, the publicity about skin cancer resulting from ozone depletion has meant that, in recent years, anxious patients have flocked to doctors with a wide range of minor skin blemishes. Most people regard cancer as very serious; some, if they suspect it, may even be too frightened to go to the doctor. Particularly sad examples of this, which are unfortunately not uncommon, are the older woman with a slowly growing fungating carcinoma of the breast or the young man with a treatable testicular growth.

4   Patients weigh up the advantages and disadvantages of taking a particular course of action. They do not necessarily take all the relevant factors into consideration, but feel able to make an evaluation. (*Perceived costs and benefits.*)

This cost benefit analysis is unique to every individual and can be influenced by outsiders, including doctors. However, for the doctor to be able to influence the equation in the patient's favour, they need to know which factors have already been included. Think about Mrs Arthur and her fears about treatment. Her fear that radiation would prevent her conceiving might stop her from complying with the treatment because, in her mind, the risks of treatment outweigh the benefits. The doctor needs to seek out such fears and talk them through with the patient.

5   Patients' beliefs do not already exist prepackaged. They are prompted or created by a number of stimuli and triggers (*cues to action*), such as physical sensation, what Granny said, a television programme or what has just happened to the man down the road.

The health belief model emphasizes what we have already discussed. People are generally engaged in a struggle to understand what is happening to them and what might happen. A person's belief system is unique but strongly influenced by race, culture, religion and their immediate society. A poor Chinese peasant will have a very different understanding of health from a German banker, but so will people living in the same environment. There will be little similarity between the understanding of health of a Geordie miner and a black Rastafarian living in Newcastle. There are major differences in different strata of the same society and differences are even considerable within the same social group.

The health belief model threw up another concept — *locus of control*. This is jargon for how we explain to ourselves what is likely to happen to our health. Using this idea we can divide the human race into three types of people.

The internal controller

This type of person believes that fundamentally they are in charge of their own future health. In other words, what happens to their health is largely the result of their own actions. This is the muesli eating, brown rice and leather sandal brigade who digest every morsel of health-related news from *The Guardian* or *The Telegraph* health page. It is the type who will not have an aluminium pot in the house for fear of Alzheimer's and who are to be found sweating in health food shops rummaging for the elixir of life, having just jogged five miles to get there. There are certain implications for this type of believer, not least being that they tend to get angry if they do become ill. To spend 20 years abstaining from the good things in life to keep one's cholesterol below 5 mmol/l and then have a coronary at 55 results in a very unhappy and disillusioned human being.

As far as communication is concerned, this type of person likes explanations, dialogue and Socratic discourse. They want to be involved in decisions about their health and they want to know. The medical arguments and explanations do not necessarily need to be rational; this group are enthusiastic about alternative medicine and, let's face it, a great many medical explanations are at best dubious and sometimes frankly wrong, but if they are convincing, the internal controller will accept them.

The external controller

This character is the opposite to the internal controller. They do not believe they have any control over their health and have a fatalistic approach. The 'bullet with my name on' sort of person who can be found in the pub expounding on how the healthy diet, high fibre, lots of exercise, low alcohol theories much beloved by the medical profession are rubbish. 'My grandfather lived to be 95 and he smoked 10 large King Edward cigars a day, washed down with a bottle of Martell. He had clotted cream with everything and was shot in bed with his 25 year old mistress by her jealous husband . . . etc'.

In my career the most explicit external controller I have met was a fortyish, unfit mechanic with an expanding paunch who was complaining of being rather run down. Among other things, I gently enquired about exercise and his proclivity towards it. He knew immediately what I was trying to say.

> 'You're not talking about jogging are you doc? I'm not for that at all. Look, I reckon in this life God gives you a certain number of heartbeats and I'm buggered if I'm wasting any of mine running round in bloody circles on wet Sunday mornings!'

An external controller is not keen on Socratic dialogue, or at least not as far as their health is concerned. They want to be told what to do and then to ignore the advice or not as the case may be. They are not interested in involvement and take little or no interest in the media's obsession with health. Curiously, research in this field suggests that people with an external locus of control are more likely to be influenced by the simplistic and vast poster campaigns much practised by well-intentioned organizations like the Health Education Authority, exhorting people to avoid a variety of pleasurable but possibly dangerous activities.

Most important for us to remember is that the form of communication that works best with the internal controller will not work with the external controller. Now we come to the third type of person.

The powerful other

This type is quite different from the others. They do not believe that they are in control of their own health nor are they fatalists. They believe **you** are in charge of their health.

> 'I have this terrible cough doctor. I know it's not related to my smoking because I've been smoking for a long time and it has never bothered me. I would like you to give me something to stop it.'

Doctors, of course, see a disproportionate number of this type of person. The patients described as being 'heartsink patients' are mainly to be found in this category.

Powerful others pose another difficult challenge for us as doctors. Strategies for trying to persuade such patients to take more responsibility for their own health are firmly resisted. Getting them involved in deciding how to proceed is also difficult as powerful others are quite firm about their agenda for the doctor and are happy with authoritarian doctors who relieve them of any responsibility for their own health. They are not easily educated, and if their ideas and intentions regarding their own health do not coincide with their doctor's, they will not follow the doctor's advice.

Influencing locus of control

The good thing about locus of control as far as doctors are concerned is that it can be influenced. It is rather like a political affiliation; most of us lean to the left or right, but can be cajoled sometimes into voting the other way. Locus of control in most people is a tendency, not a fixed aspect of their personality. A further point about external and internal beliefs about health matters is that we are not necessarily consistent. For example, I may be quite a fatalist at heart, but I still buy Volvos, believing them to be safer for my family, and perhaps for me. If it is correct that the communication strategy of the medical profession should be directed towards encouraging people to look after their own health and taking some responsibility for their health, and I believe it should, only the internal controllers are going to accept this idea easily. The other 50–60% of patients are going to need some persuading. However, the effort may be worthwhile for several reasons, not least because it is likely to lead to more patients following more medical advice.

One last thought in this chapter. If patients all require different styles of communication, depending on their locus of control, and research suggests that doctors have on balance fairly inflexible styles, how are we, as doctors, going to develop the necessary flexibility without spending all our lives at communication workshops? Heaven forbid.

The answer must be to explore our patient's agendas. If we understand their beliefs, and have an inkling about their locus of control, we can try to follow at least some of their agenda and talk to them about what matters to them and us. Communication will, therefore, become tailored to the individual and automatically become more flexible.

CHAPTER 4

The patient's learning circle

David Pendleton first demonstrated this idea to me in 1980, and we describe in detail the patient's cycle of care in the book *The Consultation. An approach to learning and teaching*. What follows is a slightly idiosyncratic version of that original description.

When patients meet doctors and some form of communication takes place, they are changed. Not necessarily in the ways that doctors may hope for or expect, but some change in understanding occurs. It is important for us to analyse the effects that our contacts with our patients have on their subsequent behaviour and beliefs about health and illness.

In the previous chapters we have thought about some of the issues which affect patients' decisions to consult and what the factors are which make up their health understanding. It is now time to consider the role of doctors as educators in this learning circle. Let us start with the outcomes.

Commitment to plan

When a patient has consulted you, they come away having made immediate decisions about whether to follow your advice or not. There are

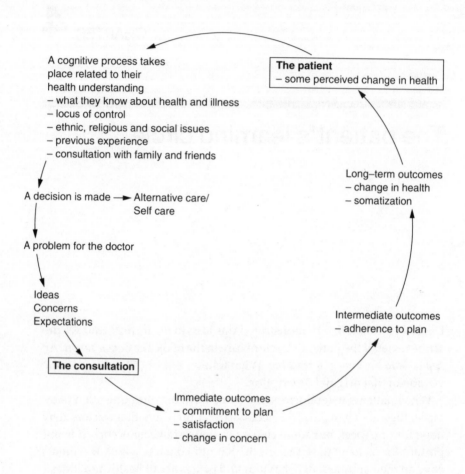

A cognitive process takes
place related to their
health understanding
– what they know about health and illness
– locus of control
– ethnic, religious and social issues
– previous experience
– consultation with family and friends

A decision is made ──► Alternative care/
Self care

A problem for the doctor

Ideas
Concerns
Expectations

The consultation

Immediate outcomes
– commitment to plan
– satisfaction
– change in concern

The patient
– some perceived change in health

Long–term outcomes
– change in health
– somatization

Intermediate outcomes
– adherence to plan

Figure 4.1: The patient's learning circle.

many reasons why they may follow your advice. The first and the best is that they believe and understand you and that their agenda is close to yours. Other reasons include doing what one is told by a respected professional. This may result in the idea that it was not quite what they were expecting, but you are the doctor so they will try it. Or they may just be too frightened to disobey.

The problem is that more than 50 per cent do not follow our advice. They are not committed to the plan, probably because it is your plan, not theirs.

For example, a 54-year-old man is referred to the cardiology clinic by his GP with a letter saying 'This man has developed intermittent chest pain over the last 3/12 which has some cardiac features such as being related to exercise and radiating to his left arm. His resting ECG is normal, BP 150/85, and I cannot find anything obviously wrong. He smokes 20 a day and is a line worker at the car plant. There is no past history of anything significant'.

The clinic is rushed as usual, but you take his history in more detail and examine him thoroughly. You think, like the GP, that there may be an element of angina and you arrange for him to return for a treadmill test and give him some GTN tablets to put under his tongue when the pain begins. Later you hear he defaulted on the treadmill test. Why did he default?

In this case, the reason was simple. He thought you and his GP were investigating the wrong thing. He went to his GP with chest pains, worried that they heralded the onset of oesophageal cancer because his father had presented in the same way. The thought that the pain might be related to his heart had occurred to him, but it did not correspond to his idea of heart pain. He was confused that his GP did not mention cancer or ask him about his throat, but he was worried that his GP really did think it was cancer because he sent him to hospital. He kept his appointment because he thought the hospital would carry out tests which would rule out cancer. When he found out that you at the hospital were, like his GP, only interested in his heart, he did not feel committed to your plan. He presumed you were not worried about cancer. He was not worried about his heart, so he decided to do nothing unless something else developed, in which case he would go back to his GP.

Change in concern

The immediate thought that most us have is that going to a doctor will reduce a patient's concerns. However, this is of course not true. Let us take a simple headache as an example.

In the town in which I work, probably 100 people wake up each morning with a headache, and one or two come to the doctor. They usually, but not always, turn out to be the most concerned out of the hundred.

The first is a woman of 25 who is afraid of her recurrent headaches, thinking she probably has a brain tumour. She is hoping to be taken seriously and properly investigated and treated. She has come today because it is particularly bad, and she had a row with her boyfriend last night about a TV programme about doctors misdiagnosing cancers. I am rushed and although I do not discover all this, I do discover her fear of a brain tumour and see her immense relief at being allowed to talk about it. I examine her thoroughly including her fundi. This is, of course, supposed to be both diagnostic and therapeutic. After discussion, explanation, advice and the offer of a possible follow-up appointment, she leaves with less concern than when she arrived. Her health understanding has changed a little, but the change is brittle and it will not take much to bring her back.

Our second patient is a 56-year-old banker who says he is not too concerned about the recent onset of migraines because his mother began to suffer from them at about the same age, but he would like some of those new injections or something like that which he read about in the evening paper. We go through the same routine; this time I notice a nystagmus to the left and papilloedema of the left disc with a fuzzy right disc. He picks up on my concern, and the urgent need for a neurological opinion raises his anxiety level considerably.

This is a rare event in general practice; most headaches are not caused by brain tumours. This example is intended to illustrate the rather obvious point that concern can increase after a successful consultation. This point, although not subtle, needs to be borne in mind when reading learned papers about changes in concern.

To go back to Mrs Arthur in the first chapter, when she first went to her GP, he examined her thyroid thoroughly and did a blood test; he did not mention cancer and neither did she. Did he not mention it because he thought it was cancer and did not want to frighten her? Was the blood test for cancer? He did say something about going to hospital. Was that to see a cancer specialist? She was not less concerned on leaving.

Remember the interchange at the hospital. How do you think her concern changed? If she is very concerned about possible I131 treatment, and nothing you have said has alleviated this concern, then her health understanding will remain unchanged and she is likely to default.

The effect that the doctor's style can have on the patient's concern is worth repeating. Respected authoritarian physicians have the power to reduce anxiety at the cost of reducing patient autonomy and this effect is sometimes shortlived. However, giving ill patients too much autonomy can raise anxiety. This is a difficult equation and deserves your attention. Sharing information and understanding would seem to be the best compromise as being most likely to increase autonomy while constraining any increase in concern.

The last point about concern relates to a curve well known and much loved by psychologists (*see* Figure 4.2).

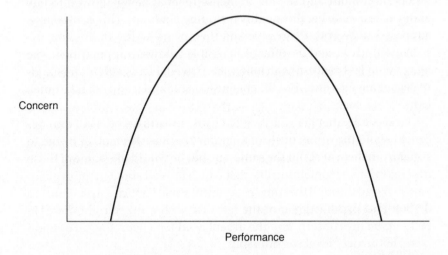

Concern

Performance

Figure 4.2: Concern measured against performance.

As you can see, performance increases with concern to a certain point and then plateaus and falls off. This curve should interest doctors too. If the anxiety or concern is too great, patients will not do what it is in their best interests to do. This may be why showing rotting cancerous lungs in bottles to smokers is not usually a very effective technique for helping them to give up. It pushes the majority over the top of the curve. Too great a fear of cancer freezes patients into inertia, whereas a small decrease in concern may put them on peak performance to enable them to face the rigours of the treatment. This is a simple but very important curve. Keep it in mind.

Satisfaction

This is a commonly measured factor in many articles about doctor/ patient communication. The simple equation is high satisfaction = good, low satisfaction = bad. However, as usual, life is not quite that straightforward. Many health messages are not particularly satisfying, even if a jury of peers would concur with them. The current craze for lifestyle advice is an obvious example. The patient comes to her doctor with a cough and is told to stop smoking, lose weight, have her cervix smeared, her breasts examined and cholesterol measured, and is then told that the doctor cannot prescribe her with any cough mixture. To a large section of the community this may be profoundly unsatisfying, but to the majority of the profession this would probably be seen as good practice. (The author would probably abstain if a vote were taken.)

There is an easy way of satisfying most patients, and that is to give them what they want. Most alternative therapies work on this principle. The fact that patients often want treatments such as unnecessary antibiotics, excessive time, more of you than you can spare, dubious operations etc means that the goal of only satisfying patients is a poor one. We need more integrity than that. Again, it becomes obvious that patient satisfaction is a subtle measure and needs careful interpretation.

Intermediate outcomes

Compliance

There is a difference between the 'commitment to plan', immediate decisions about compliance and the full follow through to complete the course. Defaulting can occur at any of these stages. The poor uptake of medical advice remains a major challenge to our profession, but it could be argued that within many patients' health understanding there lurks a health scepticism related to medical advice, and that if we, as doctors, really do wish to influence our patients to do what we think is good for them, we had better be jolly certain that we are right.

The patient will usually comply if they understand and believe the explanation. Some will comply because it is a doctor who has told them to; most will comply if their understanding seems to match that of the doctor and their agenda is shared. A shared understanding should be a general professional goal.

There is a fascinating area that doctors know very little about — what lessons do our patients learn from whether they follow our advice or not?

Ninety-nine per cent of patients act rationally in terms of their own health beliefs which, however, may not themselves be rational. For example, Patient A goes to the doctor wanting penicillin for her sore throat, she gets it, gets better and has her health belief confirmed — that penicillin cures sore throats. Patient B does exactly the same, but does not get better — what lessons has he learned? That pencillin does not

	Patient gets well	Patient does not get well
Patient complies	A	B
Patient does not comply	C	D

Figure 4.3: The effect of compliance on understanding.

cure sore throats? That it was not a 'strong' enough antibiotic and the doctor was ineffective in choosing the right one? That the doctor was right all the time and it was a virus that did not respond to penicillin. That there may be something very serious that the doctor has missed? That this doctor is no good and that he will try another one next time? etc. There is another possibility with Patient B — that of partial compliance. He might be one of the one third of patients that take a few pills here and there but not enough to get adequate blood levels (but he may think he has followed instructions).

What about Patient C? He only came for a sick note, but was given tablets he did not want, did not take and he got better. Or Patient D? She was given penicillin but did not take it because it had given her thrush last time, but now she feels both unwell and guilty. These are just some of the examples of the sorts of messages that patients relate to whether they do or do not take our advice. How many of these sorts of messages are we aware of?

Let us go back to Mrs Arthur and put her in each of these boxes; and assume that she has a borderline toxic goitre.

In Box A, treatment with I131 is agreed upon, her fears about fertility are dispelled and she complies with the treatment that is unpleasant but that she has been prepared for. She feels a little better and is grateful for your attention. She still worries about the lumps but is now more likely to accept any further recommendations, such as an operation.

In Box B, she has an unpleasant reaction to the treatment and feels quite poorly. She is totally unprepared having had little or no explanation of what the treatment entails, and she is horrified that she had to stay in a little side ward away from everyone else and that even her husband was only allowed to see her through a leaded hatch. She is convinced more than ever that she will be infertile and she wonders if you have made an incorrect diagnosis or if your management might be wrong. She is not happy with the hospital and may default on any further follow-up.

In Box C, she refuses to come for I131 treatment because of her fears. Anyway, she feels fine now and she thinks that you ordered a dangerous and unnecessary treatment and she has little faith in your opinion that she does/does not need an operation.

In Box D, she refuses to come for I131 treatment for the same reasons as in Box C, but finds herself losing more and more weight, and she becomes frightened and afraid of calling her own GP because she has not followed medical advice.

Of course, the changing course of her illness could easily move her from box to box, constantly altering what she is learning from these experiences; her health understanding will also be changed by each meeting with her doctor and by the outcomes of these meetings.

Whether or not the patient complies, leads to the final outcome in the patient's learning circle.

Long term effects

Change in health

We all try to make sense of changes in our health, and tend to link them to changes that preceded them. For example, a patient with a bad cold may come to believe that a large tot of Glen Morangie is the best solution if improvement follows in the morning. A patient may quickly come to believe that antibiotics cure colds if the doctor prescribes them with little explanation. Both of these learned beliefs can be seen as superstitious and neither is helpful for the patient or doctor. Look again at Figure 4.3 — what other superstitions can patients develop?

Somatization

This final outcome of the consultation is an area which doctors are just beginning to pay attention to. The word is ugly and obscure, but means the tendency of patients to create physical symptoms out of emotional responses; this can be aided and abetted by doctors strenuously trying to create a disease out of a mass of complaints, and a disease created in a patient's mind is very hard to dispel.

Look again at the patient's learning circle (Figure 4.1) — in what areas are your interventions likely to influence your patient's health understanding? Remember that your chance to influence this understanding may not come very often (particularly if your patient is a young or middle-aged man).

CHAPTER 5

The doctor's circle of understanding

This is, of course, the other side of the patient's circle, meeting at the consultation. There is, however, a big difference between the two. Most patients do not go round the circle very often; doctors are going round all the time. I saw around 6000 patients last year. I wonder how many I learned from? We are often told about learning from experience. Most doctors quite quickly have a lot of experiences with patients, but how much do they learn from these experiences?

The doctor's circle of understanding can be drawn as follows (*see* Figure 5.1).

Physical and emotional status

How we feel affects how we consult. If you have 'flu and still find yourself at work, it can be very hard to think straight and to make decisions, and when it is apparent that most patients are feeling better than you are, some of your motivation will evaporate. It is obvious that doctors consult better when they are well, but many doctors, driven by inner goals, soldier on long after the point when it would be better for their patients if they stopped.

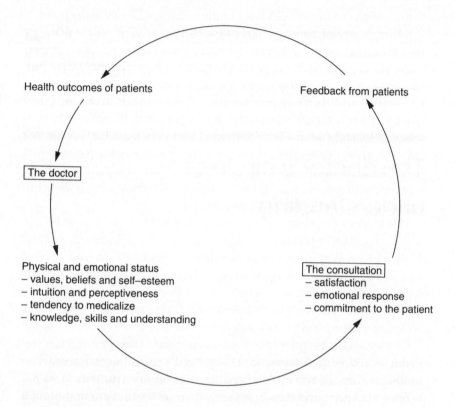

Figure 5.1: The doctor's learning circle.

Emotional health is more subtle and more insidious. Doctors have a very high incidence of alcoholism, depressive illness and chronic stress disorders. The stiff upper lip, lonely, evangelistic, medical credo forces them to carry on against the odds, rarely seeking help from colleagues as this is perceived as a sign of weakness. However, at last the profession is beginning to wake up to the emotional needs of doctors. If you feel yourself becoming emotionally stressed, talk about it with friends and seek help sooner rather than later.

Values, beliefs, attitudes and self-esteem

Like patients, we bring to our consultations a set of beliefs, moral values and attitudes which are derived from our own upbringing, culture and experience. These thinking and feeling patterns will influence how we consult with our patients. A few simple examples illustrate the point.

If I am an atheist, I am less likely to suggest to a dying patient that they seek solace in God. If I believe in the total sanctity of human life, I am virtually never going to recommend a termination of pregnancy or to be involved in discussions about euthanasia. If I am politically left of centre, free market health service policies may be an anathema to me and I may work in a way which demonstrates my disapproval. If I believe that unsolicited lifestyle advice is an intrusion into personal liberty, I am not going to give it very often. If I believe that it is better for patients that they should be protected from the whole truth in serious illness, then I will withhold information. If I believe that the patient's ideas and concerns are important, then I will seek them out, etc.

Think about your own beliefs and attitudes. How do they affect the way you consult or feel about patients? Can you compromise from time to time? Can you justify your attitudes to yourself? To your peers? Would you say that you have an accepting attitude in relation to your patient's point of view and beliefs, or is it more a judgemental attitude which equates your patient's worth with their knowledge and beliefs and places your point of view above theirs?

Our self-esteem is relevant. What is our status? How important is status to us and how motivating? Do we need to be powerful in order to protect our fragile self-esteem? Do you consult with patients in such a way as to enhance your own self-esteem, or is this not too important a factor to you? How important is the approval of your friends and peers? How do you maintain your self-respect when dealing with your patients? How do you develop self-confidence? Think about it.

Intuition and perceptiveness

This is both God-given and learned. Intuitive medical behaviour may be based on experience — an effective synaptic short circuit — but some doctors are better at it than others. Usually the more intuitive are the more experienced doctors. When you are learning, do not trust too much to intuition. Go back, re-check, try to trace the intuitive pathway until you can follow a logical thread.

Perceptiveness must be learned. Sherlock Holmes remains one of the finest role models, based by Conan Doyle on a senior medical figure in Edinburgh. Consulting with patients, looking, asking and examining them form the basis for developing your perceptive skills. Really seeing them, truly hearing what they say (or do not say) and understanding them and their context enhance them further. Later in the book are some exercises to help develop your perceptiveness (*see* page 57).

Tendency to 'medicalize'

Ivan Illich coined this deliberately ugly word to describe the medical tendency to organize vague symptoms into categories, labelling these categories and so producing a disease which can then be approached in the traditional medical manner. This tendency is particularly obvious in the medical handling of the everyday emotional trauma which all human beings experience. For example, unhappiness is a human condition, whereas 'depression' is a disease that can be treated with anti-depressants. Labelling people creates illness; people found to have mild hypertension and told this fact, suddenly have more sickness absence, a higher incidence of impotence and see themselves differently. There is also the medicalization of daily living; encouraging people to consult doctors for the minor vagaries of life and health, a creeping stripping of personal autonomy, the gradual creation of a society dependent on the medical professions for all wisdom on diet, exercise, lovemaking and everyday existence.

If we as doctors subscribe consciously or unconsciously to this widespread tendency, it will affect the way we consult and the outcomes of those consultations. A medicalizing doctor and a somatizing patient are a bad combination.

Knowledge, skills and understanding

This is the area traditionally related to the medical school. It is for the knowledge, and the skills to use that knowledge, that the public come to us. We learn about diseases and techniques to diagnose and treat these diseases, we listen to aphorisms like 'There is nothing more important than diagnosis, diagnosis and diagnosis'. We slave over sweet-smelling corpses searching for aberrant nerves, and learn by rote the mysteries of the Kreb's cycle. We are multiple-choiced to the point of exhaustion and we are taught to learn by an adversarial style of oneupmanship. We feel guilty about reading a novel because we should be reading medicine. There is so much it is unencompassable, and if we are not careful, in all this knowledge we lose our understanding of people and what makes them tick.

We must use our consultations with our patients to increase our knowledge, to hone our skills and, most of all, to improve our understanding of illness, of people and of ourselves. Then, with all these strands of ourselves mixed together as our 'givens', we come to the consultation, there is an interaction, a conversation, some laying on of hands — whatever — but at the end of the consultation some things have changed for us like they have for our patients. Let us look at these possible outcomes.

Satisfaction

We all want to do a good job and to take pride in doing so. It affects how we perform. For instance, there is some evidence which shows that doctors who have low job satisfaction prescribe more tranquillizers and antibiotics, and have shorter consultations. In order to get regular satisfaction from patient encounters, we need to like what we are doing, have reasonably clearly defined aims and get frequent, supportive feedback to tell us how we are doing and how we can improve. I suspect that not many of us get much of that sort of feedback.

Satisfaction also relates to several internalized goals and measurement of our achievements against these goals.

> 'That was a good consultation. She came in
> very unhappy, but I spotted that. I let her cry
> and then she told me what was really worrying
> her.'

The goal is to increase your perceptiveness in order to increase your therapeutic potential.

> 'That was a good consultation because I diag-
> nosed myxoedema.'

The goal is to be a good diagnostician. 'I was satisfied with that consultation because I felt we really did achieve a genuine shared understanding.' etc. Think about some of your own goals in dealing with patients. From what do you derive satisfaction?

Emotional responses

Dealing with people who are seeking your counsel can be immensely rewarding if your knowledge and skills enable you to help them. This can give you a buzz, an emotional high, unmatched by most other occupations. There is a downside too. You will meet many you cannot help very much, some in great distress; some you will meet and know from the start that the outcome is only a lingering, painful death. This is hard for you and you need to develop strategies to cope with this emotional pain. Many doctors do this by retreating behind cold, professional veneers, sharing little with their patients, telling them less, effectively switching off. There are more effective and less dramatic stategies than these. Helping people to die can be very gratifying if done well, especially with patients whom you have got to know as people. There is emotional pain, but tempered by the satisfaction of helping a fellow human being through those last days, weeks or months. Sharing knowledge, showing compassion, alleviating pain, facilitating communication with spouses and family, using other medical skills to maintain tolerable bodily functions to the end and not deserting them. Unless you specialize in terminal care, most doctors do not see dying patients very frequently, so there is no need to develop armour plated communication techniques. In the vernacular 'stay loose'.

There are myriads of possible emotional responses to a consultation. Sad people may make us sad. Michael Balint suggested that the way patients make us feel is a pretty good guide to how they are feeling, so if you are angry at the end of a consultation, maybe your patient was angry too. Consulting under time pressure, as most of us do, creates its own stresses and frustrations. In a busy clinic, when you are already an hour late, nice Mrs Jones trying to tell you her life story can wind up your innermost spring until your teeth clamp together.

There are also those especially difficult patients, usually frequent attenders with incurable problems, demanding that you do something for them. This group have been labelled 'heartsink'. Most clinics have at least one patient in this category. Somehow you will have to learn how to retain a sense of humour, of compassion and to keep too much cynicism at bay. It is true that looking at the list of patients to be seen can, on occasions, produce a pre-consultation gloom. This is one advantage of reaching consultant status; you can pass on such people to your juniors.

Roger Neighbour, in his illuminating book *The Inner Consultation*, discusses ways in which doctors can care for themselves. He calls it 'housekeeping', the point being that unless we can keep ourselves in good trim emotionally, we cease to be effective with our patients, and our personal lives can suffer. You should read this book.

Commitment to the patient

After a consultation, some sort of bond has been formed. It may be tenuous and fragile, or it may be a true contract with responsibilities on both sides. There has to be some commitment on our part or we fail as carers. Our patients certainly expect us to follow through and to be involved with them. In our learning circle, we will experience many different levels of commitment. Here are a few examples:

- The terminally ill young wife with advanced breast cancer. You have become very involved with her and her bewildered husband, so much so that you have given them your home phone number to call at any time. Now that is commitment.

- The pleasant, but chronically anxious schoolteacher with increasing panic attacks. He rings you when you are very busy and asks to see you as soon as possible. You offer him some time when you should be off duty. More commitment.

- There is Mrs Arthur holed up having her iodine treatment. She sends a message asking you to come and talk to her. Do you go? She asks you to contact her husband and explain to him what is happening. Will you?

We cannot commit ourselves deeply to all patients we come into contact with. We would be swamped. But we must give each of them a degree of commitment. It is part of our learning circle to judge the appropriate level of commitment we need to make to an individual who seeks our help.

Feedback

The feedback we receive from our patients is haphazard and highly selected. The happy ones come back, write us letters, send us occasional presents, tell us how good we are and make us feel good about ourselves. The patients with whom we have been less successful may never come back; they will probably not contact us at all; we may rarely be chastened and hear one of them discussing us in unflattering terms on top of a bus, but usually we just do not hear. This means that feedback from patients is very distorted in our favour. It is easy to spend one's life in a fool's paradise.

Doctors need unbiased constructive feedback. We are not going to get this easily from our patients so we must do it ourselves. Later in the book we will work through ways of achieving this.

Health outcomes of patients

If our patient gets better thanks to our ministrations, that feeds back into our knowledge store, as does the patient who does not get better. On a mechanistic level we can learn from our various tinkerings what helps and what does not. We often pretend to be academic, but most doctors will trust their own experience of 10 people on a particular drug than a clinical trial of 1000. 'I have seen it before and know that that happens' is a traditional part of the art of medicine. This is not to deride the scientific basis of some of our knowledge, or to belittle the power of the double blind randomized controlled trial; it is just to acknowledge human behaviour and the power of personal experience.

Every patient is unique and this is why medicine is so hard to teach and to learn. What works for one will not work for another. If we observe carefully the outcomes and develop our perception, this will feed back into both our knowledge and understanding store and increase our intuitiveness. What we have to take into account of in this equation is not just the treatment we gave, or the advice we proffered. We need to remember the style in which the consultation was conducted; whether it was doctor-centred, patient-centred, relaxed, rushed, how the relationship was etc, as all these factors will affect what happens to our patients.

Look again at the full learning circle (*see* Figure 5.1, page 32) and think of five recent patients you have seen. Write down what the outcomes of those consultations were for you and then think how those outcomes feed back into your 'givens', the items listed before the consultation.

OK? Done that? Then now it is time to look into the black box to see what the consultation should contain. Read on MacDuff.

CHAPTER 6

What you need to achieve in a consultation

What follows is not the same as the traditional method of history taking. In some ways it amounts to the same thing, but it is a better method. The concepts are rooted in the discussions in the previous chapters and the model works for all consultations in whatever setting. There are five tasks and several subdivisions of each. Here they are:

- discover the reasons for a patient's attendance
- define the clinical problem(s)
- address the patient's problem(s)
- explain the problem(s) to the patient
- make effective use of the consultation.

To use an American expression, let us 'unpack' each task in turn.

Discover the reasons for a patient's attendance

Before you started reading this book, it may have seemed obvious in most outpatient clinics why most patients were there. Now I hope it is apparent to you that patients do not come to doctors because they have liver disease; they come because they perceive that their health has changed, and they have a whole set of beliefs and expectations relating to this change in health. On the whole, it is doctors who tell them they have liver disease. So where should we start? The best bet is usually with the patient.

Listen to the patient describing the symptom(s)

You need to elicit the patient's own account of the symptom(s) which made him/her come to see you. The simplest way to do this is to let the patient talk, actively encouraging their contribution to the consultation, and watching them all the time. Look for cues — verbal, non-verbal — try not to interrupt too much. Use your perceptive faculties to hear what they are saying, and try to pick up the message behind the message. We will discuss some of the effective skills later in the book, but for now just think for yourself how best you would encourage the patient.

There are good reasons for letting the patient have a minute or two of relatively uninterrupted dialogue at the beginning of a consultation. The first is that it often saves time. You were not expecting that were you? You were thinking that if you let the patient take over the consultation it will go on and on. The reasons why letting the patient talk can save time are related firstly to the patient's agenda and secondly to yours.

The patient, and only the patient, knows the reasons why they have come to you. If you start on your agenda too soon you may never discover the fear of cancer, the fear of the effects of therapy, but more importantly, you may not discover what it is that the patient actually wants to know. You may spend 30 wasted minutes testing and reassuring them about a normal cardiovascular system when their actual concern is oesophageal cancer. The woman with the breast lump who returns following a positive biopsy needs to tell you her ideas, her fears, her expectations to help you both to plan the best management.

The point about you starting on your agenda too soon is significant. It is well documented that doctors make hypotheses very early in a consultation, usually in the first 30 seconds, sometimes even earlier. Once you have made a hypothesis, for example, 'This woman has toxic multinodular goitre' all your energies are channelled in to proving that hypothesis. There follows a rapid fire series of clinical, closed questions directed towards that end, to the exclusion of a broader picture. Another hypothesis will only arise if your clinical search is sterile. You will gain so much more valuable information by consciously delaying making your first hypothesis for, say, just one minute. Try it.

At all times keep watching your patient, so that you do not miss any cues, verbal or visual. You do not always have to act on them, but ignoring patients' cues will mean that you will be less effective. Here are a couple of examples:

At the end of your history taking with Mrs Arthur in outpatients you ask 'Is there anything else worrying you?' to which she replies 'Er . . . . . . no I don't think so', while dropping her gaze and nervously fiddling with her handbag. Do you take this denial at face value or do you pick up on her verbal and visual cues and perhaps say 'There is something isn't there? Try to tell me what is worrying you.' Later while examining her, you ask about previous pregnancies and she says that she has no children, but you notice that her eyes moisten and there is a slight catch in her voice. Do you ignore these cues? Or do you say something like 'You seem a little upset, why is that?' or 'Is becoming pregnant something very important to you?'

Obtain relevant social and occupational information

Why not do this at the beginning too? At least you can then place your patient in a social context and begin to know a little of them as sentient human beings with homes to go to and, if they are lucky, jobs to do. You will need to elicit sufficient details to place the complaint(s) in a social and psychological context, and perhaps to gain some knowledge of the cause(s) of the problem.

You will also need to establish the effect of the illness on work or home life. Doctors often forget about the effects, but to our patients these may be the main reason for them coming to us. A chain smoking miner with advanced emphysema may be hoping for some more breath to allow him to walk to the Club and to be able to climb the stairs to visit his disabled daughter. The fact that we may not be able to offer him more breath but know his reasons for coming to us, may help us and him to make a realistic assessment. We can then offer the help of other agencies for wheelchairs, stair lifts etc while not pretending that we can perform any magic.

Explore the patient's health understanding

If you have let the patient talk for a while, some of their understanding will have been revealed, but some will need actively searching for, their ideas, their fears and concerns, and their expectations. Remember Chapter 3. You might get an inkling about their locus of control. This in turn may help you choose a more appropriate style of communicating. You must take the patient's health understanding into account in enough detail to ensure that there is a reasonable probability that the consultation will be successful.

Enquire about other problems

The presenting complaint may not be the most important to the patient or to you. The patient may be presenting with an acute complaint while also suffering from a chronic condition. An acute pneumonia in a diabetic, intermittent claudication in a patient on beta blockers for hypertension, thyrotoxicosis in a woman with multiple sclerosis etc. You must obtain enough information to assess whether a continuing complaint represents an issue which must be addressed in this consultation.

Now to the 'proper' doctor bit.

Define the clinical problem(s)

Having discovered, in the patient's words, why they have come, you can now form a working hypothesis and start to put some of your clinical pigeonhole skills into operation.

Obtain additional information about critical symptoms or details of medical history

Firstly, you must obtain sufficient information to be sure that you are unlikely to miss any life-threatening condition. Secondly, your verbal investigation should be consistent with your hypothesis, which you have now formed on the basis of information obtained in the consultation. This part is well taught at medical school, but do observe how your chiefs consult. What history taking shortcuts do they use? You may have to learn how to 'take' a full history but there will be few times in your career when you do not modify what you have learned to be more appropriate to the circumstances.

Assess the condition of the patient by physical examination if appropriate

The examination you choose should be one likely to confirm or refute your hypothesis or any other hypothesis that could reasonably have been formed on the evidence you have so far. This can be a little difficult, as the more experienced and expert you become, the more hypotheses you will be able to generate. A thorough and intelligent examination is required. This next sentence may sound like heresy but — whisper it quietly — some patients only need examining to reassure them, to address a specific concern. For example, take an anxious young woman with intermittent chest pains. The power of the examination and negative ECG is almost always therapeutic, not diagnostic. Most good physicians are aware that if they do not know the diagnosis after talking to the patient, the examination rarely illuminates.

Make a working diagnosis

In primary care, detailed clinical diagnoses are uncommon in the sense of the widely used disease model of medicine. The diagnosis becomes a flexible concept to allow the formulation of a rational and appropriate management plan. For example, sore red throat for three days,? Strep? Virus, patient not ill and not too fussed about antibiotics, just needs reassurance. Or, recurrent headache with all the characteristics of tension in a chronically anxious frequent attender who will need some strategy or therapy to improve these headaches.

In hospital, the disease-based formulation is more dominant, but dangerously exclusive as already demonstrated. For example, multinodular goitre with hot spots, needs more investigation and probably surgery.

Doctors need to form clinically appropriate working diagnoses on which we can formulate further plans for refinement of the diagnosis if necessary, or on which to base a management plan for our patient.

Address the patient's problem(s)

Assess the severity of the presenting problem

You have to use some judgement here. The simplest example is triage, practised by battlefield surgeons and casualty officers on Saturday nights. You will have to divide your patient's problems into types with differing degrees of severity and then treat the individual problem appropriately. On a battlefield you would not treat a man with toothache, in casualty you treat the life-threatening condition before all else. In outpatients, the patient with long-standing irritable bowel who is cachectic with a knobbly liver needs rapid investigation for malignant disease, and in general practice the woman who presents with a sore throat, mentions her chilblains and only later casually mentions a slightly lumpy neck needs you to consider her multinodular thyroid gland in some depth.

Choose an appropriate form of management

Your management plan needs to be appropriate to your working diagnosis. This is part of the knowledge and skills taught at medical school and modified by experience throughout your career. Your management should of course reflect a good understanding of modern medical practice.

Involve the patient in the management plan to the appropriate extent

Patients should be involved in choosing their own management plan as much as possible, not least because their co-operation will be needed for the plan to be implemented. Management options should be shared with patients and where appropriate the patient should make the choice. You may initially find this concept uncomfortable, but it is likely to make you more effective and less prone to 'medicalize'. Encouraging patients to see themselves as responsible for their own health may alter their locus of control a little and make them more likely to request information, as well as to use the medical profession more appropriately.

Explain the problem(s) to the patient

Share your findings with the patient

You must always try to explain your working diagnosis, what management options seem appropriate and what the possible effects of any treatment are likely to be.

Tailor the explanation to the needs of the patient

By now you have got to know your patient a little. You should have a feel for the sort of person they are, so that when you begin to explain, you should ensure that your manner and language are appropriate to the patient's needs and presented in terms which they are likely to understand. A common medical fault from the highest to the low is to cloud explanations with technical medical jargon incomprehensible to almost everyone. Do not do it.

Your explanation should be linked to the patient's beliefs which you have already elicited. This does not mean that you have to adopt all your patient's beliefs; some may be quite erroneous, but you must tailor your explanation specifically for them. This will make it much more relevant than the standard talk on hysterectomy or the routine explanation about irritable bowels.

Ensure that the explanation is understood and accepted by the patient

Doctors, on balance, are quite good at giving explanations. The fly in the ointment is that patients are bad at understanding them. Watch your peers explaining to patients and ask yourself whether they are explaining for their patient's benefit or their own. Many explanations by doctors appear to be given to make the doctor feel that they have completed their own consulting process and that the patient is barely relevant. Ask yourself, am I explaining for me or for my patient?

What you must do is to explain your diagnosis, your shared management plan and the possible side-effects of treatment. Even this is not enough. You must keep checking with your patient that they understand you. This is a skilful process and we will touch on it again later, but be warned that a glassy eyed passive patient nodding obediently is not necessarily grasping every pearl of wisdom that falls from your lips. You must make some attempt to reconcile your viewpoint with that of your patient. What you are trying to achieve is a *shared understanding* and this is different from a simple explanation. An explanation is a one way process. I am the full vessel and I will pour my knowledge into the empty vessel that is my patient. This does not work, it has to be a two way process.

Make effective use of the consultation

Make efficient use of resources

Time
Perhaps the most precious resource of all is time. As Richard II said, 'I

wasted time and now doth time waste me'. We must make efficient and sensible use of available time and, if necessary, recommend further consultations as appropriate. The use of time by doctors is a subtle area of study. It is not the length that is so important, but the use to which the time is put. In general practice, it probably takes a minimum of 10 minutes to achieve a reasonable degree of shared management and shared understanding. It probably takes longer in outpatient clinics as you usually do not know the patient. The examination is likely to be more protracted and you may have to confer with your chiefs. In the USA, paramedics see the patient prior to the consultation with the doctor, and often very comprehensive questionnaires are completed that can short circuit or facilitate the gathering of information, if used as an aid to communication. In some of the clinics I have attended, sadly, they often acted as a substitute.

Investigations

Any investigations that you order should be capable of confirming or excluding the working diagnosis. There should be no place for armfuls of blood to satisfy every whim of the senior registrar. Costs are important and should be justified in terms of the refinements any results might make to the overall management of the patient. If a test will not make any difference to the outcome or the management of a particular case, it must be very hard to justify. Always ask yourself why am I doing this test? Will it clarify, confirm or refute what I suspect? Is it really necessary?

Other (health) professionals

You must consider the possible involvement of other professionals, such as nurses, physiotherapists, other medical specialists etc. Only make referrals when necessary and appropriate as decided in the management plan agreed with the patient.

Prescribing

The cost of drugs is forever escalating and the burden on national resources of inappropriate, uneconomical and unused drugs is enormous. Whenever you prescribe, ask yourself these questions: 'Is this the best choice of drug for the condition?' 'Could I get the same efficacy more economically?' and 'Will my patient take them?'

Establish an effective relationship with the patient

The word 'effective' is fundamental here. What you wish to achieve is a relationship which helps you to complete the other tasks. You must discover the reasons for a patient's attendance, define the clinical problem, address the patient's problem, clearly explain and make overall effective use of the consultation. How you achieve this is your business. You may well have been taught interpersonal skills such as empathizing, eye contact, use of touch etc. These are all very well but, if used unthinkingly, may just produce clones of slightly damp Methodist ministers who are just too warm and hold your hand for five seconds too long (apologies to Methodists but I had to upset someone). We have all met lovely, warm, empathetic doctors who are frankly ineffective, and also come across some pretty unpleasant, cold fish who are effective. It almost does not matter if you consult in green spotted pyjamas wearing a goofy hat, if you can regularly achieve a shared management plan and a shared understanding. It is the achievement that matters not the means of getting there.

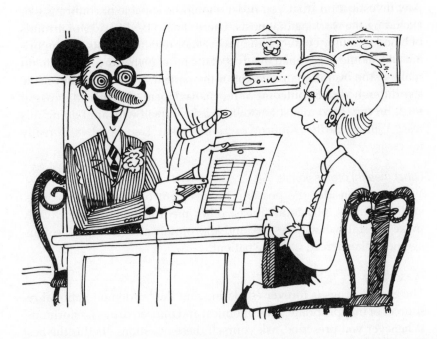

I am exaggerating, but not a lot. There are of course some styles of behaviour which are more likely to result in an effective relationship than others, not least a genuine show of interest in your patient as a fellow human being, but there is no one style that will suit all. Concentrate on your strengths, what you feel comfortable with and work on your effectiveness. If you are consistently failing to achieve an effective relationship with patients, then some of the analytical methods discussed later may help you to diagnose your problem and help you find an appropriate remedy.

Give opportunistic health promotion advice

There are some areas of preventive behaviour which doctors as a profession are pretty convinced of, such as smoking is bad for you, immunization is good, as is regular moderate exercise, probably regular cervical smears etc. Other dietary and lifestyle messages depend on your beliefs; such as the value of regular breast self-examination, cholesterol watching, egg eating and salmonella, and the legions of other advice in the 'Nanny knows best' style. You have to make the best decisions you can on the available evidence. The point at issue here is, do you use an appropriate moment in the consultation to give such advice? Linking lifestyle advice to a current illness can be quite an effective way of altering behaviour. Simply telling patients to stop smoking and giving them a leaflet will mean that 5–10% will give up, an astonishingly high figure if you think of how many patients you see. This is another area for you to think about. The consultation does provide the opportunity for such advice, but not to the exclusion of the patient's agenda.

CHAPTER 7

Ways of looking at the consultation

The first problem with looking at your own communication with your patients is that you have to *want* to do it. Nobody wants to look at their inept, stumbling and wooden performances do they? I mean why wear a hair shirt unless you are a monk? Life is just too short. Well, to begin with you must; you owe it to your patients and, what is more, if you learn to look properly, you will find it fascinating, illuminating and immensely rewarding.

Creating a climate for learning

Looking at yourself consulting is unnerving initially. Others looking at you can be terrifying. Why is this? There are several reasons. There is the fear of being found wanting, of being exposed, of being attacked and ridiculed. There are certain taboos in our society about what you cannot criticize, car driving and lovemaking being the two most obvious examples. Consulting could be a third.

Our medical school training often does not help; we are used to a point-scoring, adversarial, oneupmanship style of teaching. You have to know one more syndrome than your colleague, think of the blood test no one else has thought of, and take pretty fierce criticism on the chin. Some years ago, a young nervous student was having the mysteries of a diabetic retinitis demonstrated by an aggressive and impatient chief. The student had not fully grasped the skills of ophthalmoscopy, but was desperately trying to maintain some personal credibility with his irascible tutor. 'Well what do you see?' To all observing, including the chief, the ophthalmoscope light was now brightly illuminating a patch of pillow to the left of the patient's head and it was obvious that the young man was not seeing anything of the retina. Gamely, but unwisely, he continued giving a fictitious description of what he was not yet skilled enough to see. The chief bellowed at him, 'You silly little worm. If you had an IQ of one less you would be a plant . . . . . .' This form of constructive feedback is not likely to make us keen to reveal our innermost secrets to a group of doctors. So, how can we create a protected environment? Easy, just two rules.

Rules for feedback

Rule 1. Good points first; Rule 2. No criticism without recommendation.

There you are, simple eh? There is actually a third rule which is, always to obey the first two.

Simple these rules might be, but that does not mean that they are always easy to keep and enforce. Let us look at rule one first. I have worked with trainee general practitioners for several years and these rules are foreign to most of them. So after they watch their first consultation I say 'Great. OK. Now, what did you do well?' This more often than not produces a phenomenon I will call the 'Goldfish sign'. A glazed look spreads over their physiognomy and their mouth begins to open and shut involuntarily, emitting no sound. Most of us are not used to recognizing what we did well. We watch ourselves with mounting self-disgust.

> 'Oh Lord, look at that. I missed that cue altogether. Gosh, I'm glad my professor didn't see that examination. What a rotten explanation. I don't think I understood it let alone the patient. She'll never come back. I was just so awful . . . etc, and then some idiot asks what I did well! I didn't do anything well! It was all terrible! Oh God. . . . . .'

Ah, but you did. You did many things very well indeed. You may need a little practice to recognize your strengths, but recognize them you must or the baby goes out with the bath water. Learning from watching yourself consult must be a building exercise not a destruction exercise.

If you are watching with a colleague or a teacher, it seems to work best if you start the discussion. In other words, the doctor being observed should start any discussion with what they did well. It is often necessary to clear away matters of fact, but do not be sidetracked into covert criticism. 'Which drug did you prescribe?' is fine. 'Do you normally examine the chest through the shirt?' is not. If you are having difficulty in recognizing your strengths, this is when your colleague or teacher can help. No criticisms at all at this stage. Only when you have a thorough understanding of what you did well, and the skills you used to achieve your success should you move on to areas where you think you were less effective.

Doctors are very good at being critical. After all, we are not stupid. The problem is that our talent for supportive constructive criticism is often underdeveloped. There is no place for criticism without recommendation.

> 'Peter, I thought when you asked her if she was worried about cancer and she began to cry, that you might have helped her more and perhaps discovered a little more about her fear. If you had just let her cry for a few moments, perhaps touched her on the arm to show you cared, maybe asked her why she was crying instead of just carrying on a little abruptly. I wonder if you were afraid of the emotions she might release?'

This is fine. I may not agree with all the comments, but I have been given some positive suggestions about how to improve my behaviour which I can use or not, and the discussion can be an open but sensitive one, where I am not unduly threatened.

> 'Peter, you were a bit insensitive when she started to cry. You must work on that and do better next time.'

This is unhelpful because I do not know what to work on. I am just left feeling vaguely inadequate.

Start using the rules now with your friends and try to persuade some of your teachers to follow suit. In my experience of groups there is sometimes an initial frustration at the constraints imposed by these rules and someone will say in as many words 'Come on Peter, stop pussyfooting about. Hit me with what you really think. What am I bad at?' The problem with this approach is that eventually the teacher can relent and do just as requested. The result being obvious in the metaphorical sense. If you hit a human being hard enough they will always fall over, and that is what happens, and why the rules are there in the first place. Do not break them. Using such rules does not mean that you cannot touch on difficult personal areas and areas of special sensitivity. It just means it takes time to create a supportive trusting environment where such delicate and meaningful discussions can genuinely take place to the considerable benefit of the learner, you.

Ways of looking

You do not need high-tech equipment to look at how you consult. For a start, thinking over what you have just achieved with a patient is something. Being observed by a colleague who can give you supportive feedback helps, and all that needs is an extra chair. Psychotherapy departments are prone to one way mirrors, although I must confess to never feeling comfortable with such a set up. The disadvantage with all those methods is that there is no action replay. The advantage is that patient consent, although it should always be asked for, does not need to be formalized.

The two methods of recording most in use at present are audiotape and videotape; laser discs are on the horizon. Audiotaping is cheap, unobtrusive, easy but pretty boring. Videotaping is much more stimulating. You catch the expressions, the non-verbal behaviour and it is just more likely to hold your attention. However, it is more complicated, harder to set up, more threatening and there is more to go wrong. Having said all that, most families have used a camcorder at some stage and the technology is familiar. Modern equipment is low-light sensitive, and will work in the dingiest of outpatient suites or surgeries. It is all colour these days and most equipment will date, and more usefully, time stamp the tape. There are a variety of formats which can be confusing, the large and lesser used full size VHS being the most useful as it allows four/eight hours of recording on one tape. The smaller more convenient camcorders have restricted recording times which can mean that the tape runs out in the middle of a crucial consultation, but this is likely to improve.

The on camera microphones are now quite good but if you want good sound quality, and it is poor sound quality that ruins more tapes than anything else, you should use an external microphone. Many hospitals have audio-visual departments that can help, and most general practice trainers have experience of regular videotaping. Equipment can be hired in any high street and can be bought for less than £600, still a tidy sum but it can be used both personally and professionally. Many general practices now have fixed camera brackets in surgeries, but most will need a tripod. A wide angle lens helps a lot, as many consulting areas are pretty cramped; although you can simply double the focal length bouncing off a mirror, you lose light, but modern cameras are so light sensitive that this does not matter. The intention must be to have patient and doctor in shot with clear facial expressions; if you can only get one clearly, go for the patient.

Simulated patients

If you ever get the opportunity to work with actors or health professionals simulating real patients, do take it. You can get real feedback from an articulate non-passive patient telling you what they really thought about your strengths and less effective strategies. The wonderful thing about simulation, as a learning tool, is the fact that in real life it is almost impossible to know what any patient's 'script' is. In simulation this is known, so you can see how far you got.

Simulation is also very useful in short-circuiting your learning circle, being able to produce particular patients with particular problems on demand. There are groups of actors, in the UK and particularly in the USA, specializing in realistic simulation of patients. In the States, some actors have developed the facility to simulate real physical signs such as peritonitis, and even tenderness of the cervix simulating ectopic pregnancy! This may well be a growth area in medical training.

Role play

Role play is do-it-yourself simulation and can be very useful. Unfortunately, most people come out in a rash as soon as it is mentioned and cannot be found for days. It has always seemed to me that this fear is misplaced because, as long as the rules are strictly enforced, role play has some safety valves built in to it. The first is, that it is artificial and that is a legitimate defence for erratic performance, especially early on. The second is, we all vary in our ability to act and being a rotten actor is not synonymous with poor medicine, the opposite also applies. The enormous strength of role play is the occasion when you play the patient. Here you can really put yourself into their role and begin to understand what it feels like. This is worth much embarrassment and angst. Another advantage of role play is that it requires no technology but a video record does improve the usefulness.

Real patients

On balance, most people do not mind being observed, discussed or videotaped, but there have to be rules and respect for the individual. Patients know when they go to hospital that they will be seen more often than not by at least two doctors, and often by a pack. This is no excuse at all for the time-honoured medical practice of then discussing a fellow human being as if they were an antique clock with the occasional excruciatingly patronizing aside. Patients should be involved as much as possible in discussions about their condition. Detailed, jargon-ridden speculation should be continued outside their hearing. If any form of recording is to be made of the interview, written permission should be sought. The patient should opt in not out, and have an opportunity to opt out afterwards. Videotapes and audiotapes should be erased after the teaching session and if required for a larger presentation, the patient's written permission should be sought again, preferably after allowing the patient to hear or to see the recording. A sample consent form is included in Appendix 1 (*see* page 103).

Patients are less passive in the less frightening and more familiar general practice setting, and more likely to assert themselves by refusing permission to be observed. There are many studies on refusal rates (which vary from 1% to 60%), and the variables that seem to be most important, other than the patient, are the ambience of the practice and the way the message is sold. A gruff receptionist telling a new patient, 'Dr Tate is filming tonight, but you don't have to have it' is likely to elicit a much higher refusal rate than a patient who has been told when she booked an appointment that the surgery was videotaping for internal teaching purposes. Especially if she is given a leaflet on arrival offering further explanation, including assurance that any personal examination would not be on camera. Curiously, the actual condition, including problems with naughty bits etc, does not consistently explain patient refusal. It is better to get permission sorted out outside the consulting

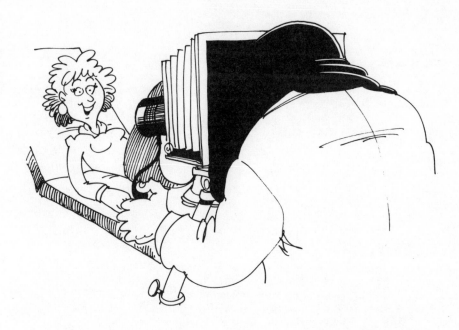

room in order to ensure that the dynamics are not too upset. Patients do not worry too much about being observed and it does not change their behaviour in any significant way. In my own surgery I had a moderately conspicuous camera *in situ* for some months, always switched off of course, without explicit permission, and only one person commented in all that time. This was a young woman requiring an internal examination who, in a compromising position, suddenly spotted the camera and said demurely, 'Do I smile now?'

CHAPTER 8

Ways of describing consultations

It is easy to discuss a recently observed consultation. There is usually some hot topic to which the conversation is drawn — often diagnosis or treatment or some patient peculiarity — but it can increase the learning potential of any observed consultation to work from a written description of the interaction. This can also then provide a hard copy of an ephemeral event. Such a description enables any subsequent ratings or judgements to be closely based on reality rather than the imperfect memory of distorted perception. I recommend three methods.

1. Mapping the consultation

A map of a consultation is just as it sounds; like a road map it can tell you where you have been, how you got there and where you could have gone. There are many types of event which can be mapped — interactions, questions, explanations, tasks etc. The original description of mapping consulation tasks is contained in the book *The Consultation. An approach to learning and teaching*. The map that I will demonstrate is similar, but based on the tasks described in Chapter 6.

The example shown is the map of the last consultation on a Friday evening (*see* Figure 8.1). The patient is male, 58 and I do not know him very well. The detailed descriptions of the consultation later in the chapter will make it much clearer, but for the moment just look at the path of the consultation as demonstrated, and observe the movement between areas which occurs.

To use the map, watch a consultation and enter a cross every time you feel a significant exchange occurs (a blank one is supplied as Appendix 2). Sometimes you will feel that two events occur at once, such as taking a clinical history and making an examination, or writing a prescription (action taken) and talking about possible side-effects (management discussion), in which case you should put a cross in both areas. The map is not a precise tool, but it will leave you with a reasonable record of the sequence of events. If two of you complete a map of the same consultation, the differences can highlight different perceptions and form the basis for significant discussion and learning.

Many consultations, especially in general practice, contain multiple problem presentations. To distinguish these on the same map, you can use other symbols or different coloured pencils. If your videotape does not have a time stamp, you can record the video recorder index numbers at points on the map of significant interest to allow easy replay. After completion of the consultation, join all the crosses and other symbols together sequentially using a ruler. With a little practice, you can map consultations of colleagues while their consultations are in progress. This gives you a permanent record without technology and stops a lot of arguments about what did and did not occur.

Now you have your record, what use can you make of it? Firstly, you must be aware of what the map does not do very well. As I have said, it is like a road map; it will tell you the places you visited and the ones you did not, but it will not tell you what they were like. Road maps do not tell you whether it was a pretty village or an ugly, run down place — you have to make that quality judgement. Just so with the consultation map. Your map may show you spending 10 minutes on examining your patient, but you and your colleagues will have to judge how appropriate and efficient the examination was. The map only tells you that you did it, not how well you did it.

However, because of its sequential nature, a series of maps of you consulting can be very revealing. Perhaps demonstrating the 'tomorrow never comes' syndrome. This syndrome is characterized by the response to a query as to why a particular task was not performed during that consultation.

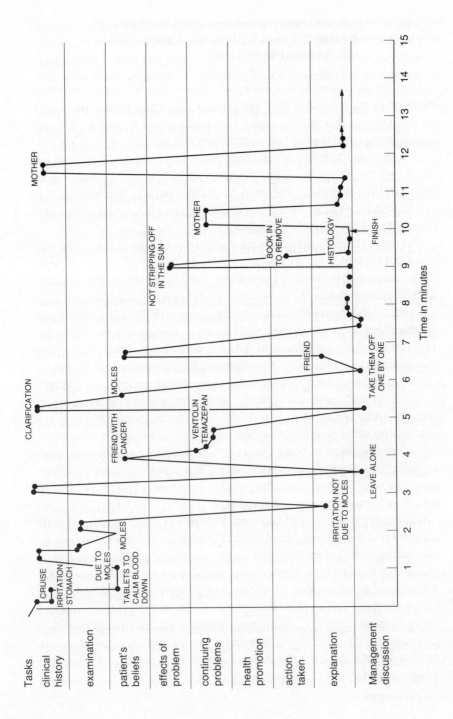

Figure 8.1: A consultation map.

'Oh yes, certainly patients' concerns are important, but I was a bit rushed this time. I will definitely ask him next time.'

A look through several more maps of your consultations may reveal none of them have an entry for patient concerns. Tomorrow never comes. Used in this way, the map provides a guide to performance by highlighting regular poor task completion.

The map will identify pivotal movements in the interchange which can then be dissected at leisure. The map as shown (*see* Figure 8.1) does not chart the relationship between doctor and patient. Not because it is not important, but because it is very difficult to be precise about and does not lend itself to this technique.

The most effective way of using the map is to have a list of the five tasks and the subdivisions, and to go through the consultation systematically measuring yourself at these tasks. Do it in silence at first and then start any discussion with the tasks which you performed well, and why you performed them well. What are the criteria which you use to decide whether they were performed well? Learn to recognize your strengths. You can use the map to help by writing notes on it at the appropriate places. Little vignettes of conversation, significant statements by one or other, what the problems were such as 'sore throat, goitre, unhappy etc'.

The map will, of course, clearly reveal tasks which were not performed. You have to ask yourself whether you can justify this. Perhaps health promotion was inappropriate, for example, but most tasks are required in most consultations if you are to be an effective doctor. Measuring your consultations against the tasks a few times will soon make you aware of your style of consulting and of what steps you may need to take to become more efficient and adept.

Look again at the example map (*see* Figure 8.1). What does it tell you? It shows that the consultation lasted 12 ½ minutes. It shows that the history taking included an examination and some of the patient's beliefs. It shows that the effects of problems did not play much part, but that there was a brief consideration of continuing problems, including the patient's mother. The explanation phase of the main problem (moles) seems to have lasted for about three minutes. The words appended to phases on the map remind us of what occurred and allow us to review quickly a particular area if it seems helpful. Look back at this example when you have read the rest of the chapter.

2. Consultation self-appraisal proforma

I am indebted to Roger Neighbour for this idea which has been developed as both a learning and an assessment tool. This method of describing the events of the consultation has to be completed afterwards and can only be completed by the participant. You can do it from a map to remind you and give you the timescale, but it is better if the consultation has been recorded and you can review it slowly, stopping frequently.

Here is how to do it followed by a completed example: review your recording (or map) of the consultation, and stop the tape after each minute of elapsed time. On the proforma describe or summarize, in not more than 40 minutes, what happens in each successive minute. Mention any significant remarks, observations, insights, thoughts, explanations or decisions. The idea behind this device is to highlight your own perceptions of what occurred and why. This tool, unlike the map, also lends itself to exploring the developing relationship between you and your patient. The following example (*see* Figure 8.2) is the same male patient of 58 as shown on the map, whom I do not know very well, but whose elderly mother I see regularly. This was the last appointment on a busy Friday evening.

As you see, this is essentially a descriptive tool, but it forces you to collect your thoughts about the events and with an astute teacher all sorts of topics can be discussed. The map and this proforma are complementary. When you get a chance to observe yourself, I would suggest mapping most consultations and filling out the proforma on one or two of the more interesting ones (a blank form is supplied as Appendix 3).

3. A workbook

This is probably a good idea at medical school and also whenever you change disciplines. It works well in general practice. The idea is to formalize some of your self-observations into a collection which you can add to as the years pass, and which will give you a measure of your own personal development. There are many items you can record in a loose-leaf workbook, but let us now concentrate on reviewing your consultations.

To complete a comprehensive review of a consultation, one more form is necessary. Figure 8.3 is an example of such a form, completed for the same patient as described above.

Time in minutes	Observations
0–1	I am tense and one hour late. He wants tablets to calm the blood down! I think he is anxious and I need to hear more. I let him talk.
1–2	He tells me of his moles. I ask a couple of questions seeking the cause of his irritation. I think he is very afraid of cancer.
2–3	He tells me more about his moles and I examine him — both a clinical and a therapeutic procedure. I tell him that moles do not cause irritation.
3–4	I continue to examine him, get some more history and now he tells me about his friend who died from a cancerous mole.
4–5	I check his medication in search of the cause of the irritation. Temazepam rears its ugly head. We both note it and continue.
5–6	I pause, tap the desk, consciously stopping in order to clarify and review where we have got to. I involve him in the management decision.
6–7	I suggest, in a long-winded way, that in view of his concerns, I will remove his moles.
7–8	He talks about his friend. He is quite frightened.
8–9	He asks me how I can tell the difference between a bad mole and a good one. I embark on an explanation.
9–10	I'm still explaining. It is rather one-sided. I do not check his understanding and ignore some verbal clues.
10–11	He tells me that for the last year he has been frightened to strip off in the sun. I tell him to make an appointment for a minor operation and tell him that the histology will confirm that all is OK.
11–12	He wants to talk about his frail mother. I am tired, reluctant to say too much, but share some of my thoughts.
12–13	He is kind to me and I feel uneasy. He lets me know that he is worried about his mother, but appreciates that there is no easy medical answer.
13–14	He leaves and I wish I had spent less time on his moles and longer on his mother.

Figure 8.2: A consultation self-appraisal proforma.

Age of patient: 58   Sex: M   Length of consultation: 13 minutes
New problem or follow up?: N   Do you know the patient?: Y
Describe the main reasons for the consultation
C/o 1. skin irritation — anxiety re moles
       2. anxiety re elderly mother.

List the outcomes of the consultation, for example prescription, referral,
no action taken, certificate, review, procedure etc.
TCI for minor operation by me next week, to remove two melanotic
lesions and one seborrhoeic wart. ? Freeze that one.

Figure 8.3: A consultation assessment form.

What did you do well?
Took him seriously. Gave him time and let him explain his anxieties. I
answered his questions with a long explanation. I knew the consultation
was really about his anxiety, the moles had no stigma of malignancy.
What would you have wished to improve on, and how?
I should have checked his understanding more. Looking at the video, he
was not taking it all in. It might have been improved if he had not had to
wait for an hour. I should have tackled his Temazepam habit, but could
not face it on that occasion. Next time!
Describe any special features of the consultation
I was an hour late, and tired. The previous consultation was emotionally
draining.
Describe any health promotion
There was not any, unless you include removing moles.
*Do you think the patient was satisfied with this consultation? Give reasons for
your opinion*
Yes. I think he was reassured and pleased with a positive decision about
his moles. He seemed grateful for the care his mother is receiving.

As you can see, with a map, a proforma and an assessment form you
have a pretty comprehensive description of a consultation and your perceptions of it. With the help of a good teacher you can also make a note
of the areas of discussion and what you learned, and keep these as a permanent record, a guide to your developing abilities.

CHAPTER 9

Useful strategies and skills

There are many skills which can be useful to doctors in particular circumstances. The skills for clinical history taking and the clinical examination are beyond the scope of this book, but here are some which relate to communication, some of which you might find helpful. Do not merely learn new skills for the sake of it; follow the diagnostic procedures described earlier in the book. Discover which skills you already possess and try out new skills in those areas in which you are having difficulty. The dreaded role play can really help when trying out and learning new skills.

Strategies and skills useful for discovering the reasons for a patient's attendance and defining the clinical problem

■ Delay making your hypothesis for one or two minutes. When you have made it, test it, but be prepared to let go easily and to form another hypothesis and yet another as necessary. Try to generate several possible hypotheses. Do not judge too quickly or by appearances.

- Ask the same question the patient has asked themselves. Why has this patient come? Why now? What has happened? Why has it happened? Why to him/her?

- Search for the patient's beliefs, ideas, concerns, expectations, feelings and the effects of these. Try to allow the patient to voice his/her real concerns.

- Use your general and specific systems enquiry sensibly and in a discriminating way.

- Examine thoroughly but appropriately.

- Put the patient at ease, lessen their anxiety and try to encourage them over their natural diffidence.

General skills for good interpersonal communication

- Listen with genuine interest.

- Actively encourage the other person to talk.

- Show understanding and empathy.

Skills for assessing the patient's mental state

- Look for the *minimal cues*. Watch your patient carefully and listen to what they say. You must practise true seeing and hearing.
  - Watch their facial expression, where they look, what gestures they make. Do they make eye contact? Watch their posture, muscle tone, breathing. Do they look anxious, sad, angry? Think about their dress, general appearance. What might Sherlock Holmes have deduced?
  - Listen to them carefully. What does their speech tell you? What are they not saying? How are they saying it? Too fast, high pitched, too slow, normal rhythm and modulation? Professor Higgins remarked that the moment one Englishman opened his mouth, another Englishman despised him. We learn a lot the moment our patients say something, regional and ethnic accents being immediately obvious. We obtain further clues about our patients' internal thought patterns by listening to their vocabulary, figures of speech, metaphors, imagery and their deletions, distortions and generalizations. Let me enlarge on the last three.
    A *deletion* means some detail(s) essential to a complete under-

standing is missed out by the patient. For example, 'I feel worse'. Worse than what? In what way? 'The whole lot are worried about Gramps.' Who in particular? How worried? About what in particular?

A *distortion* means turning actual behaviour and events into protective abstract concepts which have a reality of their own. For example, 'I just lost my cool'. What is cool? It does not mean you can shout and swear at the receptionist. 'I'm suffering from my nerves.' What does that mean? That you want more valium, to see a psychiatrist or that the weekly trip to the supermarket is now a nightmare due to increasing agoraphobia?

A *generalization* means arguing from the particular to the general in a manner which excludes any possible exception to the rule they have made. For example, 'I hate doctors'. All doctors, all the time, me? or 'I'm always getting headaches'. Every week, month, day?

Roger Neighbour's book *The Inner Consultation* deals with these areas, and related skills, in more detail.

- Learn to recognize the patient's *internal search*, and do not interrupt. You need to notice when you have asked the patient a question which they were not expecting or when a chance remark of yours makes them stop and think. Give them time to think; do not continue with your own agenda until they are ready.

Skills for eliciting

- Speak the patient's language. Do not talk down to them and avoid jargon.

- Remember that, at the beginning, the patient is always right.

- Let the patient go first.

- Make statements which make good questions. For example, 'I was wondering whether....', 'Sometimes I find....', 'It occurred to me that....', 'My friend John.....', 'Some people.....', 'I've known cases where......' 'I had a patient once.....'

- Ask open questions; they are good for finding out about patients' beliefs. They cannot be answered with yes or no. For example, 'Would you tell me about....?', 'What is it like?', 'What are you worried about?'

- Ask closed questions which are good for obtaining and classifying facts and for pattern recognition. They are bad for eliciting beliefs and feelings, they tend to increase doctor control and they can only be answered very specifically, often with only yes or no. For example, 'Is it painful?', 'Are your waterworks all right?' (one of the worst medical euphemisms!).

- Give encouragement such as 'Go on'. Eye contact and nodding encourage patients to continue. If you find that your patients will not stop talking, you may be fixing them with your gaze and nodding benignly, transmitting the message that you wish them to continue talking. Echoing is a good technique for encouraging patients to continue their narrative. This means repeating the last few words of their sentence when they pause, to encourage further revelations.

- Check what they have said. This can be done by giving them your interpretation of their story, enabling them to correct any misunderstanding and embellish the story further.

- Explain why you are asking a question. This can stimulate unexpected responses. 'The reason I asked about wind and bloating was that I was wondering about irritable bowel syndrome.' 'Oh, my sister's got that and she said that's what I've got, but my GP reckons it's an ulcer.'

- Use silence. This is often frightening to young doctors who, every time there is a pause, feel uncomfortable and duty bound to say something, however inane. Try allowing pauses. The patient will invariably fill them if you wait long enough.

Strategies for addressing the patient's problem

- Negotiate with the patient.
- Influence the patient and involve them in the decision making.
  - Counter your patient's fallacious arguments and erroneous beliefs.
  - Reinforce those beliefs that are helpful to the outcome.
- Try to foster patient autonomy and increase patient self-reliance.
- Use your power carefully (*see* Chapter 2). For example, should you sit behind the desk instead of to one side, fill your room with potentially frightening medical paraphernalia, etc? Do not let your personal attitudes intrude too much.

- Be prepared to admit uncertainty.

Strategies for getting the patient to do what is good for them

- Make things easy. People are more likely to do things if there are fewer things to do, if they fit their existing lifestyle and if they have the necessary resources.

- Think of the context. People are likely to do things if they do them with other people, if they are reminded at the time to do them, if they know someone might be likely to check to see if they have done them and if the people with whom they live and work are willing to help them.

- Think of the patient's perceptions. People are more likely to do things which seem important, and when they understand why they should do them and how to do them. If they really believe in your advice, they will follow it, and they are more likely to do things if their anxiety level is raised moderately but not too high.

- Think of the relationship. People are more likely to do things if they have helped to decide what would be beneficial, if they have promised to do them and if they have faith in you as their doctor, especially if they think that you like and respect them, and they are more likely to do things if they are rewarded for doing them.

Negotiating skills

- The doctor goes first.

- Think aloud, and state your position. Be honest. Give the patient a few choices.

- Ask the patient what they think. Reinforce the patient's good ideas, counter the bad ones.

- Watch their internal search. If you do not see the patient looking as though they accept what you say, continue to negotiate. Watch for 'non verbal leakage'. This may sound like a pool of muddy water forming around your patient, but is actually the discrepancy between what your patient says and what their non-verbal behaviour is indicating. For example: 'No, I'm not depressed', while sitting with shoulders slumped, a sad fixed expression and exuding gloom. Or, 'Yes, I will probably try the tablets', while breaking eye contact and squirming in the chair.

Influencing skills

- Not saying 'Don't' unless you mean do. For example, 'Don't worry' means that worrying is an option. 'Won't' means might, 'Can't' means could and 'Shouldn't' means probably will.

- Use questions as statements. For example, 'Do you ever think you'll come off the tranquillizers?'

- Use shepherding techniques. For example, use value laden phrases to direct, such as calling an osteopath 'a bloke that tweaks backs for £20 a time' or 'a colleague with more training in manipulation than me'. Or using presuppositions such as 'Do you think you will find it easier to stop smoking all at once, or gradually cut down over a fortnight?' Or use the 'My friend John' technique such as 'I remember someone else who did what you are thinking of and found out the hard way'.

- Use appropriate delivery, that is how you say something, not what you say. Break information down into manageable segments. Keep pausing and checking. Is the patient following what you are saying? Pace — the speed of delivery — is important. Try to match the patient's rate of speech. Eye contact is important. Keep watching for those minimal cues. Try to match the patient's language of self-expression.

- Reframe statements/questions and alter the perspective. For example, a three-year-old boy who is brought in because he 'wilfully' scratched his baby sister's face, could easily be labelled 'attention-seeking' which could make things worse. What if he were labelled 'attention-needing'.

Strategies for explaining and achieving shared understanding

- Elicit the patient's beliefs. You cannot share unless you have something to share.

- Recognize that the whole consultation, particularly the process of eliciting, organizing and reflecting the information the patient gives you, is an experience from which the patient can learn.

- Translate and share your medical knowledge honestly and with respect for the patient.

- Maintain or enhance the patient's autonomy.

- Be prepared to admit uncertainty.

- Clarify how much information your patient wants.

- Do not reassure too soon. This can be interpreted as rejection or a lack of knowledge.

Explaining skills

- Present information without using jargon, but using short words and sentences as specifically as possible.

- Remember that the order information is given in is important. Patients recall best what they are told first.

- Repeat important pieces of information.

- Provide explicit categorization. For example, 'I am going to tell you what I think is wrong, what I expect to happen and which treatment I suggest'.

- Use leaflets, tapes, laser discs, Healthline etc.

- Encourage feedback and regularly check understanding.

- Do not give too much information.

Skills for sharing understanding

- Climb down a few steps from your pedestal, ie try not to be too distanced from your patient because of your need to be professional.

- Use similar phrases to the patient and some of their own descriptions.

- Share a little of you from time to time. For example, 'I had an operation once'. 'Migraines are bloody awful, aren't they?'

- Show understanding and empathy. Empathy is a much abused concept, the idea being to identify mutually with the patient and so fully comprehend them. This is fine as long as you remember that it is intended to help you; it is impossible to empathize fully with someone. How can I — a fat, white, middle-aged GP — really empathize with a young Black on crack? I can sympathize with him, I can care for him, but who am I kidding that I can empathize with him?

■ Be prepared to back down. Achieving a shared understanding does not mean getting the patient always to agree with you; it means that to achieve a genuine sharing you may have to agree with them.

■ Keep a dialogue going. You cannot share with a monologue.

■ Use all the skills mentioned earlier to discover why the patient is there.

Strategies for making effective use of the consultation

■ Determine the reasons for the patient's attendance at the outset.

■ Determine the patient's own ideas, concerns and expectations before attempting an explanation, so reducing the risk of a 'dysfunctional' consultation.

■ Use each consultation as part of a learning circle. Some tasks can be achieved over a series of consultations. The adoption of these methods may also change the patient's expectations about the appropriate use of time and resources.

■ Record information, both clinical and patient centred, effectively.

■ Obtain as much information as possible on the availability of resources.

■ Do not prescribe prematurely, expensively or inappropriately.

■ Keep the treatment as simple as possible.

■ Do nothing as much as possible.

Skills helpful in making effective use of the consultation

■ All those listed so far. To use time effectively all these skills need practising and honing. Self-observation is essential and peer observation very helpful.

■ Skills of practice and hospital management. These are outside the scope of this book, but very important.

■ Skills of appropriate control. For example, judicious use of doctor authority to control speech flow, the appropriate use of negative non-verbal behaviour (not looking at the patient will tend to staunch the flow). Closing the notes can signal the end of the consultation. Wearing a dinner jacket tends to speed patients up, but cannot be used too often. Standing up and holding the door open will stop all but the most dedicatedly self-obsessed. Taking the chair away is a last resort.

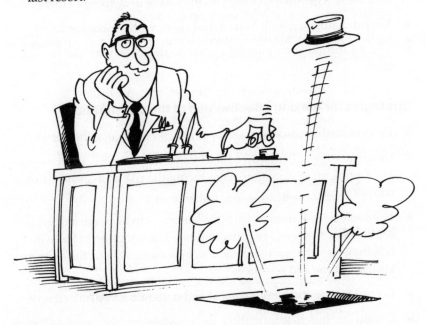

Strategies and skills helpful in relationship building

■ At the strategic level you, the doctor, should strive to create an environment that facilitates the exchange of information, for example waiting time, seating position, dress, decor etc.

■ Be friendly and attentive, adopt an informal style.

■ Use plural pronouns to indicate partnership. 'I hope you agree. Shall *we* meet again in two weeks' time, to see how you are getting on?'

■ Use self-disclosure to establish trust and common ground. 'Yes, I know you must be frightened, I'm terrified of the dentist.'

■ Make comments that are provisional rather than dogmatic. 'I think your blood pressure needs treatment, here's a leaflet to read. I would like you to come back to discuss the treatment, and what you think about it, next week.' Rather than, 'Your blood pressure is up. Take these tablets, the nurse will explain.'

- Respond descriptively not evaluatively. For example, 'What about my knees, doctor?' 'I think you have some wear and tear, possibly a little early arthritis' is OK. 'You're too fat and that's why you have painful knees' is a bit bald, dress up the message.

- Make comments that are related to the problem(s) and not related to controlling the patient. For example:

> 'I think that since your heart attack, your heart has been under a little bit of strain. You will feel better with some fluid tablets but you will need some time off work so that your heart can recover. I will make an appointment for some rehabilitation treatment which will help you get back to work more quickly. Here is a leaflet which will help explain what I mean.'

This is better than

> 'You must stay off work until I tell you. Go for rehabilitation treatment, this will be good for you and here are some water tablets to take every morning.'

- Learn to recognize the effect of your own behaviour on your patient. Are you frightening? Do you inspire trust? Do your patients come back to you? What do they tell you about yourself?

- Learn to recognize, interpret and use your feelings. You are feeling uneasy and anxious. Is your patient feeling that way too? You are getting angry, are they?

- Learn to recognize and deal with your own stress. Read Samuel Shem's *The House of God*. Talk to your friends and yourself (but not too much of the latter!). Read the section on 'Housekeeping' in *The Inner Consultation*.

Helpful strategies and skills when using desktop computers and taking notes

- Computer screens should be visible to the patient and a focus for sharing information.

- Note writing and data entry should be kept to a minimum while the patient is present.

- Read the notes before the consultation and write them up afterwards.

- The computer is only a tool —do not let it dictate the agenda.

- Share understanding and clarify the story by using and discussing the information on the screen together.

- Never enter onto the computer or your notes information you would not want the patient to see. Remember that patients have right of access to their notes and any data held about them on the computer.

CHAPTER 10

Informed consent and other ethical issues

Informed consent and other ethical issues

Informed consent is a relatively new and transatlantic concept, having first been mentioned in a Californian Supreme Court in 1957. There is no doubt that in our society the idea of informed consent is very important, very necessary and relates fundamentally to the ability of the medical profession to communicate well with patients. A brief return to the history of communication in medicine will indicate what a new idea it is.

The most influential figure in shaping the relationship between doctor and patient over the last 3000 years has probably been Hippocrates. His famous, but rather weird, oath makes no reference at all to a doctor's duty to converse with patients; in fact, in Decorum he admonishes doctors to 'perform their duties calmly and adroitly concealing most things from the patient. . . .revealing nothing of the patient's future or present condition.' Plato, in several of his writings, stated quite categorically that doctors had a right to employ lies for good and noble purposes. This Greek ethic was derived from the best of motives; it was thought to be necessary, as the belief was that without respect for medical authority there could be no cure. The idea of the patient participating in the decision-making process was seen as counter-productive. The doctor knew best. The doctor knew what was best for the patient. The main tenets of Greco-Roman medicine were that patients must honour doctors for they received their authority from God; patients must have faith in their doctors and must promise obedience. After being around for so long such ideas do not quickly disappear. How many doctors do you know who still hold views like these?

In the 18th and 19th centuries, a few isolated luminaries suggested educating and involving patients. John Gregory, Professor of Medicine at Edinburgh was a notable example, and Benjamin Rush a famous American contemporary of Gregory's held similar views but, like Gregory favoured deception whenever enlightenment was not equal to the task. They were both essentially pragmatists, seeking the most effective doctor-patient relationship for therapeutic ends and not so very concerned with educating patients to share the burdens of decision making.

Some patients were beginning to get a little restless by the middle of the last century. John Stuart Mill, the famous libertarian, put it quite succinctly in 1859, 'Over himself, his own body and mind, the individual is sovereign'. It took another hundred years for this idea to permeate through to a significant number of members of the medical profession.

Today the informed consent industry is a growth area, but the product is often pretty shoddy. Many doctors still think telling patients too much is bad for them, despite much evidence to the contrary. In fact, contrary to many doctors' beliefs, patients actually become less anxious if adequately informed about major surgical procedures, nasty invasive tests, unpleasant treatments and dangerous drugs.

The American researchers Greenfield and Kaplan turned this conundrum on its head. They asked themselves the question, if doctors do not inform patients very well, what will happen if we teach patients to ask searching questions of their doctors and to negotiate decisions relating to their own care? The references to this work are in the reading list at the end of this book (*see* page 109), but the gist of it is that they took three groups of patients from a Californian hospital — people with peptic ulcers, people with hypertension and people with diabetes — and using a randomized technique, they split each group into two, trained one group to ask appropriate questions and negotiate decisions, and then they measured outcomes. So what happened? Lo and behold, in the experimental groups the blood sugar improved significantly, the blood pressure dropped significantly, the ulcers improved more quickly and the patients were happier and liked the involvement. If these results had been achieved by a new diabetic agent, a new ololol or new itidine, the pharmaceutical companies would be ecstatic, but all that was in fact needed was some additional two way communication.

The fact that informed consent is now such a major issue is good for patients as they are offered more information than ever before. Surgeries overflow with leaflets on every conceivable subject, hospital out-patient departments have printed sheets on most known diseases and procedures, bookshops have huge sections on health and illness, magazines, radio phone-ins, television programmes and telephone lines all devote an ever-increasing amount of coverage to health-related matters. Whether doctors like it or not, their patients are becoming more informed. There is a change in society's attitude and, although individually patients still tend towards a passive role, society expects the medical profession to educate, inform and involve their patients. True consent is increasingly seen as a right, and if this right is seen to be denied or infringed, litigation ensues more and more frequently.

British law is still somewhat unclear, but the Sidaway case in England and the Moyes case in Scotland are the most recent precedents. The law does not yet seem to require that fully informed consent is obtained in all cases, but does require that important material risks should be disclosed and that all the patient's questions are answered truthfully. As a criterion of what constitutes a material risk, the 'Bolam' principle applies which, put simply, states that a doctor should act 'in accordance with a practice accepted as proper by a body of responsible and skilled medical opinion' (Lord Diplock).

The problem is that achieving true informed consent is fraught with difficulties; most consent is a long way from being informed. Most leaflets are not very good, some are poor and some make no sense at all. A northern hospital produced a detailed leaflet on barium studies a few years ago which contained every known risk, complication and detail of preparation, but it was soon noticed that patients still asked all the old questions. A journalist given one of these leaflets, got a readability score for it and discovered that only the most intelligent one per cent of the population could understand it. The moral here is that useful information presented in an inaccessible manner is useless information. More recently, another hospital looked at consent forms for cataract patients and discovered that the print was so small that more than a third of the patients could not read them.

A standard hospital technique for obtaining informed consent is to throw information at the patient. The problem is that the information is standardized and the patient is unique; the information will mean different things to different patients depending on their health understanding. What is readily understandable to one will be incomprehensible to another. A signature on a consent form may merely mean that the patient trusts the doctors, not that they genuinely understand what is going to be done to them and what risks there may be. It may be that informed consent is already an outmoded concept, and that what should be encouraged is for patients actively to request a particular form of treatment having been adequately informed of the options. This request shifts the onus on to the patient; the consumer of health care takes responsibility for their choice. This is probably 50 years away, but a logical development.

In many areas of health care, consent is taken for granted because the obvious benefit of the intervention obviates the necessity for any dialogue. Much of the screening/prevention industry works on this premise. It is in fact nothing more than a cycle of deceit and half truths, consent fudged because true understanding is not easy even for doctors, let alone patients. Take regular breast self-examination for example, and start with the patient's point of view:

> 'Regular examination of my own breasts is a
> good idea because it will stop me from dying of
> breast cancer.'

Well, the bad news is that it won't, or not on present evidence.

> 'If I find a lump it will mean I will stay healthy
> because I will have caught it in time.'

Not true, or if it is, the difference is not great. Operating on some lumps very early may even make the prognosis worse. Some lumps metastasize early, some don't. At present we cannot tell the difference.

> 'This must be a useful thing to do because the
> doctor/nurse/magazine told me to do it.'

Really. The Chief Medical Officer did change his mind recently, but was howled down and succumbed to encouraging breast awareness instead, whatever that is.

> 'It stands to reason it must be a good idea.'

It doesn't.

> 'It makes me worry about cancer, but preven-
> tion is better than cure, isn't it?'

Not when the premise is a fallacy.

Now try it from the doctor's point of view:

'It stands to reason it must be a good idea.'

Have you looked long and hard at Wilson's criteria for screening recently?

'It can't do any harm.'

It can, not least in creating false expectations and contributing to the overvaluing of medical competence.

'I can't really tell her the truth, she wouldn't believe me.'

It would take time, but she might. Honesty should be the best policy.

'But she will think I am an uncaring nihilist and that it does not worry me what happens to her.'

If that is the case, you have not achieved any degree of shared understanding and it is still not worth perpetuating a dubious quarter truth.

Try this exercise with cervical screening, cholesterol measurement, routine private medical screening, mammography, routine colonoscopies, screening for prostate cancer etc. Ask youself how much of the consent is really informed. There is a major ethical divide between your patient coming to you for your opinion and help with their agenda, and you imposing your screening agenda on them. If you do initiate such a procedure, you should have conclusive evidence that the test is likely to alter favourably the outlook for that individual and that it is unlikely to do any physical or psychological harm. Face the issues honestly and help your patients to ask searching questions.

The real crux of the whole informed consent debate is that to obtain true informed consent requires the achievement of a *shared understanding* and a *shared management plan*. This further implies that the patient's beliefs should be known and their understanding checked effectively. The ethical imperative behind achieving a shared understanding is respect for the individual. It cannot be right to achieve an agreed plan by manipulating information in a Machiavellian manner to get the result wanted by the doctor. A good model must be one of mutual persuasion by two experts; one on medical matters and the other on their own mind and body. This implies that doctors must be prepared to allow themselves to be persuaded by their patients away from their first or second choices of action if the patient's argument is an effective, convincing and, most importantly, an informed one. Doctors are not always going to like this.

The nature of the illness, of course, affects the doctor-patient relationship and the degree of informed consent. For the sake of simplicity all serious human ailments can be divided into three types.

- Acute curable illness, characterized by sudden onset, possibly immediately life-threatening, it is unanticipated, and is caused by factors usually outside the patient's control. Diagnostic uncertainty is minimal, treatment is relatively easy in a good hospital and is standardized and effective and without it the possibility of death or permanent disability is great. Septicaemia, acute abdomen, anaphylaxis, serious arrhythmias, status asthmaticus etc being a few examples. Here the wishes of the doctor and patient are usually very similar. They both wish for life to be preserved, the illness cured, function restored, pain and suffering relieved and health regained. Consent is assumed and is uninformed until after the event.

- Critical chronic illness can also become acute, but is characteristically incurable and usually fatal. For example, multiple sclerosis, metastatic cancer, chronic cardiac failure, kidney failure, cor pulmonale etc. With these illnesses, doctors must lower their clinical expectations, restoration of function is usually impossible, but prolongation of life, relief of suffering and pain and enhancement of the patient's dignity and sense of control regarding their illness is possible. These patients must be fully informed, be party to medical decisions about their treatments and be helped to make choices about the way they might die. There is a strong case for asking all patients in this category of illness about their wishes concerning the medical management of their death.

  These questions should be asked and the answers recorded in the notes:
  — If very ill and permanently unconscious, would you wish your death to be postponed?
  — If very ill and permanently unconscious, would you want, in addition to discontinuing any other life support, food and fluids stopped?
  — Would you want to be kept alive if not terminally ill but in a persistent vegetative state?

— Would you want to be kept alive if you might recover conscious-ness but would subsequently be very brain damaged (after Culver).

In these types of illness, the medical goal of prolonging life when progressive and critical deterioration of major systems is leading to inevitable death must not be an independent and overriding aim. The patient must still participate in as much de-cision-making as possible.

■ Chronic manageable illness covers those patients who are mobile, but with chronic diseases such as hypertension, rheumatoid arth-ritis, diabetes mellitus, irritable bowel syndrome, COAD etc. In these patients fully informed consent is mandatory as should be active participation in decision-taking. This is, however, a rather disease based description, helpful in hospital but not so useful in general practice which is more concerned with the daily problems of living.

Any general practitioner who wants to be an effective doctor must be in-terested in people and not merely diseases. They must be committed to their patients' welfare, willing to search out patients' beliefs and it fol-lows that they must also be willing to listen to whatever problems the patients bring to them. This is an intensely personal form of doctoring, not seen in hospitals very often. The treatment of a disease can be largely impersonal whereas the care of a patient is entirely personal.

A last thought in this chapter. What happens when, after dialogue, mutual persuasion and argument, only a very limited shared under-standing and shared management plan can be achieved because of a major conflict of values? A very common example of this crisis of rela-tionship is when a patient requests a termination of pregnancy from a doctor with strong moral or religious views. The traditional ethical solu-tion is threefold. Firstly, the doctor may simply refuse to provide the ser-vice. Secondly, they should nevertheless refer the patient to another doctor who will provide the service. Thirdly, if a doctor willing to pro-vide the service is not available, there is a greater obligation on the first doctor to acquiesce. This third course is the most difficult. It is easy to re-commend the solution of tolerance and flexibility, but it must be recog-nized that doctors are in a more difficult situation than members of the public. Doctors cannot ignore the offensive or unusual request. We can-not ignore our patients. We must choose between complicity or rejection.

In such religious or moral issues, we should share our beliefs and value systems with our patients and attempt to provide them with arguments for our stance. If our rhetoric fails, we may in turn be persuaded by the urgency and validity of our patient's arguments. If so, we should put our religious beliefs to one side. This is probably a naïve and unrealistic view, but the welfare of our patients, in the patient's view, should outweigh our own religious or moral values. The opposing view could only be correct if universal moral truths existed, which is improbable, and if they do, as human beings, we are unlikely to know what they are.

CHAPTER 11

Special situations and patients

Breaking bad news

This is not easy to do and can be such a daunting prospect that many doctors try all sorts of diversions and strategies to avoid doing it. 'Nurses are so much better at that sort of thing' is often the excuse given. The reasons for this shying away from the task are probably primarily emotional. Causing distress in another person causes distress in ourselves. Therefore, many of us do not perform very well in this crucial area of doctor-patient communication.

Common faults in breaking bad news

- Just not doing it, and hoping someone else will pick up the pieces, such as another colleague, one of the nursing staff etc. Common methods of doing this include avoiding the patient, never seeing them alone or always being in a hurry.

- Putting off the evil hour.

> 'I think we should do some more investigations.'

- Lying, or at best being 'economical with the truth'.

> 'We took the whole breast away, and the affected glands, I am sure we took it all away.'

> 'You will soon be better after the chemotherapy.'

> 'No it's not too serious, we can cure it for you.'

- Deliberately not picking up patient cues:

> 'I seem to be fading away doctor.'

> 'Really, how are you sleeping?'

> 'The treatment is not working, is it doctor?'

> 'Well, perhaps you are a little constipated.' etc.

- Going into undertaker mode, with an excessive solemnity and aura of deepening gloom. Lying is one thing, but excessive objectivity without mitigation is just as bad.

Useful strategies to help you to break bad news to patients

- Honesty is the best policy. Never tell patients anything that you know not to be true. The truth will emerge over time and the feelings of betrayal and of being misled will surface and sour your relationship with your patient and with their family.

- Do not, however, tell the patient more than he/she wants to know.

- Take great care with prognostication. *Never* give a specific time period, it will only come back to haunt you. You will almost certainly be wrong and the effect on your patient will be depressing. Hope ebbs away and anxiety increases as the stated time approaches.

- Do not take all hope away. Find some reason to be optimistic. The condition may be terminal, but you can encourage the patient to look forward to a particular event such as a birth, or to celebrating an anniversary, or they may be hoping for a period of remission or for a peaceful pain-free death.

Useful skills to help you to break bad news to patients

- Use your eliciting skills, as in Chapter 9.

- Ask patients directly how much they know about the 'bad news'. For example, remember Mrs Arthur. Let us suppose that a thyroid scan has suggested a malignancy in one of the nodules and a biopsy has confirmed this. She comes back to you for the report and your advice on further treatment. How do you proceed? Try this sort of approach:

> 'I have been so worried doctor. What did the biopsy show?'
>
> 'Do you know why we did the biopsy?'
>
> 'Yes, to see if it's cancer. Is it doctor?'
>
> 'Yes it is. I know that sounds bad, but the outlook isn't as bad as you think. Tell me what thyroid cancer means to you.'
>
> 'Does this mean it'll spread right through me? Will I die?'
>
> 'No on both counts. We should be able to remove the gland and the cancer, and make sure it doesn't return by giving you some radiation treatment.'
>
> 'That doesn't sound very nice. Are you sure you can stop the cancer?'
>
> 'There is always a risk we can't, but you would be very unlucky. The treatment I mentioned is very effective. Would you like to speak to someone more expert than I about it?'
>
> 'Well not today. But could I bring my husband along to see you and perhaps the other doctor you just mentioned?' etc.

There is a lot more information you could give her, and she may well want it, in time; but using a patient centred approach as above enables the patient to take in only as much information with its unpleasant implications as they can cope with at a time.

- Be especially sensitive. Abrupt and brutal honesty, associated with authoritarian patient control, has no place in modern medicine. For example, Mrs Arthur again. This sort of approach is not recommended:

> 'The test shows it's cancer I am afraid. We are bringing you in tomorrow morning to have the gland out. You can't hang around when cancer is about. OK?'

You must show consideration for your patient's feelings. Allow them time to think of questions and then you must answer them, and assure them of ongoing support. It is much better if bad news can be given in the context of a continuing, supportive relationship.

Do not give bad news and then make a run for it. Sit down with your patient, take your time, try to ensure that there is someone else with the patient when you leave. You may need, with the patient's permission, to contact a spouse or close friend.

- Learn to recognize and cope with denial. We all deal with devastating news in different ways. Many people cope by using varying degrees of denial. During your career you will experience situations where you have what you consider to be a sensitive, honest chat with a patient, containing lots of information, and then at the next consultation the patient totally denies having the conversation. 'They never told me anything at the hospital.'

- It is not a good strategy to break down denial too brutally. It is there for a purpose. Respect for the individual should extend to their defence mechanisms. This does not mean we ourselves have to be a party to the denial and start encouraging unrealistic expectations. We must still reply honestly to any questions.

- Family denial is another problem more commonly encountered in general practice.

> 'Don't tell him doctor, it will kill him.'

This can lead to a tragic conspiracy of silence. The sufferer knows full well that their condition is terminal, but can't talk to their loved ones for fear of upsetting them. The loved ones in turn are so afraid of upsetting the sufferer in their last few weeks that nothing about the illness, about dying, about saying goodbye etc is discussed to the detriment of all concerned. Here I think there is a place for sensitive intervention from the doctor to try to break this pernicious circle.

I believe firmly that our responsibility is to the patient and that any responsibility to the family is secondary. In this kind of situation we should tell the relatives that we will not impose the truth on the patient, but that if the patient asks we will not lie. Often with experience and tact we can get all parties to talk reasonably openly about the future and help towards a much more rewarding death, with a normal and not exaggerated grief to follow. This facilitation of family dynamics can be one of the more satisfying processes which doctors can get involved in.

■ Use emotive words with care. Whatever cancer, tumour, growth, metastases, vegetative, malignant, thrombosis etc mean to you, it is certain they do not mean the same thing to your patient. Check understanding frequently, and remember that some people, cultures and societies have taboos relating to words like cancer. Take care.

Angry patients

This is another difficult emotional area, especially if the anger is directed towards you or one of your colleagues. Being ill can make people angry, so doctors are going to encounter a lot of anger.

Strategies for recognizing and dealing with angry patients

■ Remember that it is the patient who is angry, not you.

■ Do not leave the anger unexplored.

■ Use your own feelings. If you are feeling angry, it is very likely that the patient is too.

■ Always support your staff in the face of aggression which is really aimed at you.

Skills for defusing anger in patients

■ When you recognize anger, confrontation may help.

'You seem to be cross about something.'

'Help, you do look upset.'

'Come on, get it off your chest, what is bothering you?'

> 'You were very angry with the nurse/receptionist, why was that?'

- Acknowledge the frailties and imperfections of medical diagnosis and treatment. Again honesty remains the best policy. Perceived delay in diagnosis or treatment is a common cause of patient anger. Frankness about the nature of the delay will often defuse this.

- Acknowledge your own lack of omnipotence, and watch the effects of your own guilt feelings. If you do not bring some of these feelings into the open, your relationship may be irrevocably harmed. I visited a little girl some time ago and thought she had a mild 'flu. A few hours later my partner admitted her with acute lobar pneumonia. The parents were angry at my perceived incompetence and told my partner so, and I was angry at myself and guilty for missing the diagnosis. I went to see them, feeling rather ill at ease, after the little girl was discharged, and expressed my pleasure at her recovery and my regrets for not diagnosing the pneumonia. The mother said

> 'It was not your fault doctor, you did examine her and you can't be right all the time. It did come on pretty quickly.'

They are still my patients today.

The somatizing patient

These are the patients we find especially difficult, the 'what are you going to do about my...?' (whatever it is). They get labelled 'heartsink' in general practice, and in hospital they are very quickly 'turfed' by the senior staff to the junior. The really chronic somatizer does not have his/her notes inspected, they have them weighed. This sad, irritating and enormously time consuming state of affairs is the result of a long process of medicalization by doctors and the health industry, including alternative medicine, of essentially nervous and functional complaints made by introspective individuals with a 'powerful other' locus of control.

The problem with doctors in this context is that if patients keep pushing we will eventually do something. This could be a test, which will lead to a procedure, which can lead to an operation, which can lead to a complication, which in turn will reinforce the patient's inappropriate health-seeking behaviour.

> 'See, I was ill doctor. I'm a lot better after my triple artery graft. Now about these headaches...'

I know personally a group of patients who have had coronary artery surgery, not because their arteries were in any worse shape than most, but because they persistently kept presenting different symptoms to different doctors. This led to tests being performed which were equivocal, as tests tend to be, but the pressure for something to be done meant that in the end something was done. These patients had thick notes before and even thicker ones afterwards. So what can we as doctors do about this?

Strategies for decreasing patients' tendency to become somatically fixated and medically dependent

- Use the communication methods already described, with particular emphasis on achieving a shared understanding and shared management plan. Patients should be encouraged to take some responsibility for their own health.

- Use the traditional disease-based medical model with care. While we all need to be good diagnosticians, good efficient clinical practice demands balances — most headaches do not warrant CAT scans — investigation on demand is bad medicine, treatment on demand may be worse. We must not create disease where only poor individual coping mechanisms are the problem.

- Avoid referral if at all possible. Only when all reasonable avenues and likely diagnoses have been refuted, should a referral be made. The general practitioner's primary duty is to protect his/her patients from hospital medicine.

Hospital medicine is almost exclusively disease based, patients must be diagnosed thoroughly and possible causes ruled out. Once an anxious introspective patient gets to outpatients the die is cast, investigation is coming and all that that might entail. The fixation with the symptom will be intensified and the vicious self-reinforcing loop encouraged.

Referrals should only be made for:

- Diagnostic reasons, i.e. the further testing of a specific hypothesis, the resources for which you do not possess.

- Therapeutic purposes. If you do not want or are unable to treat a certain condition.

- For reassurance. This is the really tricky one. Even if there is no traditional disease, the modern hospital's ability to dig up some minor disorder which is essentially irrelevant and overtreat it, is formidable. This can of course lead to further referral. There is also the danger that, not unreasonably, you or your chief may ask the patient to return on the grounds that although you have drawn a blank, you may have overlooked something. Both of these situations will probably lead the patient to conclude that they were right, and that there is something wrong with their health. For example, the 42-year-old female patient with atypical chest pain who insisted on referral, has a non-specific minor anomaly in a couple of leads of the ECG. This leads to echocardiography which is essentially OK and to a treadmill test which is also essentially OK, but with a performance nearer the bottom end of the normal range than the top. This leads to a full catheterization which is essentially normal, but no-one's arteries are entirely normal, and she overhears your discussion of her essentially normal variants with rising anxiety. Her consequent release of catecholamines and irritation of previously untouched places by the catheter, produces a minor arrhythmia that you need to respond to quickly and in her eyes dramatically. Her worst fears are confirmed and the seeds of cardiac crippledom are well and truly sown.

  Reasons for referral should be explicit and the doctor who accepts the referral should, whenever possible, keep within the mandate of the referral letter.

- Try to keep the number of doctors involved with a patient to a minimum. The more doctors the more somatization.

- Keep good records. The SOAP system has merit (Subjective, Objective, Assessment and Plan).

- Communicate with your colleagues about patients you suspect of undue somatization leading to 'Dr shopping', i.e. consulting every doctor in the practice in turn for another opinion, or swapping specialists frequently.

- Write explicit and detailed referral letters. These should contain biographical details, clinical and physical symptoms and signs, the course of the complaint, your own hypotheses, previous history, important psychosocial background, and what the patient believes and wishes. There should also be a clear statement of what you are asking of your colleague, and what you wish to happen after your colleague has seen the patient.

■ Use patient diaries and other methods of self-recording to try to produce more insight and linkage between events and symptoms.

Skills for preventing and dealing with somatization

■ Use the concepts of transactional analysis. You are trying to achieve an Adult-Adult relationship, not a Parent-Child relationship. Read Eric Berne's *Games People Play*.

■ Discuss your perceptions of the patient's illness behaviour.

> 'You have been coming to see me a lot recently, and I never seem to find much wrong, what do you expect of me?'

> 'It is a year since your heart attack and you seem to be leaving everything still to your wife, it is as if you do not want to get better.'

■ Discuss the patient's methods of denial and avoidance.

> 'Every time I ask you if anything is troubling you you say to me 'nobody has a perfect life' and leave it at that, but you keep coming to me with problems that I can't really help you with. You will have to help me more before I can help you.'

> 'I know you have not been well in the last year, today it is your sinuses, last time it was your tummy pain and before that your headaches, do you think there is something worrying you underneath all this?'

> 'You are trying to blame everything on a virus but I think you are not facing the real problem of your anxiety.'

■ Try to verbalize your patient's anxiety.

> 'You are afraid it is something serious aren't you?'

> 'You seem very tense, are you frightened of something?'

> 'If you go on worrying about yourself you are going to get into a vicious circle don't you think?'

> 'You have been panicking a bit recently but nothing serious has developed, can you get any comfort from that?'

■ Use the presenting signals from the minimal cues.

> 'You seem much more anxious than normal.'

> 'It looks to me as if something is really troubling you.'

■ Describe the way your patient is trying to influence you back to them.

> 'I know you would like me to send you to see a specialist but I do not think that is necessary. I am not sure what to do next.'

> 'I think you want me to give you a pill and then expect all your troubles will be over but I don't think it is as easy as that.'

> 'The way you are behaving gives me the feeling you are saying "please help me, I do not know which way to turn", am I right?'

■ Discuss and use your own feelings.

> 'Honestly I have tried everything and I don't know where to go from here, have you any suggestions?'

> 'I am sorry but you have made me feel inadequate and unable to help you, can you help me to help you?'

■ Clarify the patient's complaint(s), to give them more insight.

> 'I think your headache is caused by the mus-

> cles in the neck going into spasm, this is why painkillers don't work very well, they don't relieve the spasm. It is probably your worrying about your Mum that caused the muscle spasm in the first place.'

- Try to avoid too much advice in these patients, any advice should be specific, i.e. to give a new approach to the problem, and it should be realistically tailored to the patient.

- Encourage the patient's internal search and encourage the patient to find their own solutions and alternative strategies.

Summary

What doctors should know about patients

In hospital

CHAPTER 12

Summary

I wonder what you have learned from this book? The message I hope you will take away is that effective communication can be learned. That it is not just God given and incapable of improvement. We can all do it better, but we have to believe that the effort is worthwhile and that the goal is an important one.

Let me summarize some of the very important messages, firstly about patients.

What doctors should know about patients

In hospital

The patient is more frightened than you are. They think that their condition is more serious than you do. Most of them want to be involved in their own treatment, and want to understand what is going to happen to them.

They have not come to you about liver or thyroid disease. They have come because of their beliefs about, their expectations of and the effects of their perceived change in health. Remember, whenever possible, to put yourself in their shoes.

Your patient is probably afraid of you. They will tend to be passive and not say very much. This does not mean they do not want to know.

Patients are just people like you. They deserve respect, they need to be informed and they need to consent. However, people are all different, they respond to a change in health in different ways, and they need individual personalized plans.

People can easily have inappropriate and unhelpful illness behaviour reinforced by poorly thought out and unexplained investigation and treatment. Patients will follow surprisingly little of your advice unless you really try.

In general practice

People want to make sense of any perceived change in their health. You may be the first person they tell that particular story to and it may not make much sense if squeezed into the 'medical model'.

People come to you for guidance, for advice and for treatment. There is no explicit contract for unsolicited intrusion in the form of overzealous lifestyle advice.

People are less informed than you think. Many procedures and screening programmes need more sharing of understanding.

What doctors should know about communication

Oscar Wilde said of England and America, that we were divided by a common language. The same could be said of doctors and patients. Most patients do not know the difference between a virus, a bacteria or an amoeba. They are all bugs. Most GPs use the virus versus bacteria argument to bolster their arguments about antibiotic prescribing. How many patients are using the same frame of reference? Peter Havelock, a GP friend, told me of the time he reviewed a videotaped consultation with a patient, an elderly man. They watched it together and at the end the old man said

> 'Yes Doc, I thought that were good, but I was just a bit unhappy about one thing. You said you were going to give me antibiotics and then at the end you didn't.'

> 'But I gave you penicillin.'

'Oh, I didn't realize thems were antibiotics.'

Patients have clear expectations of what will happen in conversations with doctors. A local radio show recently had a competition for the event you would most like to happen but would be most unlikely to happen to you. One of the winners was 'going to your doctor with a sore throat and getting antibiotics without an argument about viruses'. The potential for misunderstandings between doctors and patients is unlimited.

Out of the mass of research work on communication with patients several stark truths emerge. The amount of explanation a patient receives is directly related to his intelligence as perceived by the doctor. The lower the social class, the less explanation is offered. Yet all patients from the highest to the lowest intelligence and the brightest to the more intellectually challenged want as much information as they can assimilate and in a form that they can understand. This is a very big challenge to our profession. Patients' and doctors' perceptions of patients' problems differ from those expressed both before and after their consultations. Their perceptions also differ about the consultation itself.

Asking questions only gets you answers. This is one of the problems with traditional history taking, a method of putting communication into a straight jacket in order to maximize pattern recognition.

Doctors are likely consistently to overestimate their patient's understanding. Written information, pamphlets and leaflets are useful but poorly understood by the majority of the population. Other problems with written material are not being noticed, not being read, and not being remembered.

Doctors rarely talk to patients about the consequences of their illnesses. We do usually explain a little, but we rarely share what our patients think. Our consultations are very one sided.

To consult effectively you must search for your patient's agenda and reconcile this with your own agenda. This is a skilful process, and the outcome should be shared understanding and a shared management plan.

Let us go over again what you should seek to achieve in a consultation with a patient, in hospital or in general practice.

1   Discover the reason(s) your patient has come to see you

To do this properly you need to:

■   Elicit the patient's account of the symptom(s) which made him/her turn to you.

- Obtain relevant information about social and occupational circumstances.

- Explore your patient's health understanding.

- Enquire about other problems.

2   Define the clinical problems

- Obtain additional information about critical symptoms and details of medical history.

- Assess your patient's condition by examination if appropriate.

- Make a working diagnosis.

3   Address your patient's problem(s)

- Assess the severity of the presenting problem.

- With the patient, choose an appropriate form of management.

- Involve your patient in the management plan to the appropriate extent.

- Try to achieve a shared management plan.

4   Explain the problem(s) to your patient

- Tailor the explanation to the needs of your patient.

- Ensure the explanation is understood and accepted by your patient.

- Try to achieve a shared understanding of the problem(s).

5   Make effective use of the consultation

- Make efficient use of resources.

- Establish and maintain an effective relationship with your patient.

- Give opportunistic health advice where appropriate.

If you practise the completion of the above tasks, hone your present skills, and learn some new ones as needed, you will be a better doctor than you are now. Your patients should be happier and healthier too. Good consulting.

Sample consent form for videorecording

Ideally photocopied onto surgery/hospital headed notepaper, the form, (see over), can be filled in by the receptionist and given to the patient to sign before the consultation. The patient should be asked to reattend reception after the consultation to confirm their consent. The form should then be stored in their notes.

Name of doctor_____ Date_____ Time_____

Patient's name_____ + accompanying persons_____

- The doctor you are seeing today is making a videorecording of some of the consultations with patients.

- The videos are for learning and teaching purposes with other doctors in the practice/hospital.

- The video is *only* of you and the doctor talking together. No intimate medical examination will be done in front of the camera.

- You do not have to agree to your consultation with the doctor being recorded. If you want the camera turned off, please tell reception. *This will not cause a problem or delay your consultation.*

- The video will not be shown to any doctor outside the practice/hospital without your permission.

- The video will be erased after three months, except with your permission to keep it longer.

- You can tell the doctor to switch off the camera at any time if it concerns you.

Please would you indicate your consent to this consultation being recorded by signing below. Thank you very much for your help.

Signed_____

- If, after you have finished seeing the doctor, you are unhappy and want the recording erased, please tell reception.

- If, afterwards you are happy for the consultation to be used by the doctor for teaching purposes please sign below. Again thank you very much.

Signed_____

Consultation map

Clinical history															
Examination															
Patient's beliefs															
Effects of problem															
Continuing problems															
Health promotion															
Action taken															
Explanation															
Management discussion															
Time in minutes	1	2	3	4	5	6	7	8	9	10	11	12	13	14	15

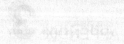

Consultation self-appraisal proforma

Time in minutes	Observations
0–1	
1–2	
2–3	
3–4	
4–5	
5–6	
6–7	
7–8	
8–9	
9–10	
10–11	
11–12	
12–13	
13–14	
14–15	

Suggested reading

Essential

Pendleton D, Schofield T, Tate P and Havelock P (1984) *The Consultation: an approach to learning and teaching.* Oxford University Press, Oxford.

This is an easy to read, if rather dry, overview of the consultation. It contains a detailed breakdown of task analyses and methods of teaching.

Neighbour R (1987) *The Inner Consultation.*

A fun book, beautifully written, that analyses the consulting process in depth. It is idiosyncratic, full of classical and Eastern quotes and immensely erudite.

Good Value

Balint M (1957) *The Doctor, his Patient and the Illness.* Tavistock Publications, London.

An ageing classic. Difficult and obscure in parts, too based on the dubious science of psychoanalysis for my wholehearted recommendation, but nevertheless the book did change general practice. The concepts of a 'drug' doctor, of 'apostolic function', of learning about one's patients from analysing one's own emotions contributed to the growth of self-respect in GPs who were suffering from low self-esteem in the 1950s and 1960s.

Byrne L and Long B (1976) *Doctors Talking to Patients.* RCGP Publications, London.

Seminal research work on what actually happens in GP consultations. The doctors' verbal behaviours are analysed in depth and the communication dissected in detail, revealing disappointing results for doctors. It is not easy to read.

Tuckett D, Boulton M, Olson C and Williams A (1985) *Meetings Between Experts.* Tavistock Publications, London.

A sort of re-run of Bryne and Long using videotape instead of audiotape. This study still showed major problems with doctor-patient communication. It is more readable.

Pendleton D and Hasler J (1983) *Doctor-patient Communication.* Academic Press, London.

Contains several interesting contributions from doctors and behavioural scientists.

McWhinney IR (1989) *A Textbook of Family Medicine.* Oxford University Press, Oxford.

The best synopsis of family medicine in print. Should be read by all doctors.

Grol R (1983) *To Heal or to Harm?* RCGP Publications, London.

An excellent Dutch dissertation on the problems with, and the prevention of, somatization.

Ley P (1988) *Communicating with Patients.* Croom Helm, London.

A comprehensive review of the research work relating to compliance with medical advice. A cautionary tale.

Of interest

Arborelius E and Bremberg S (1992) What can doctors do to achieve a successful consultation? Videotaped interviews analysed by the consultation map method. *J Fam Prac*. **9:** 61-6.

Becker M *et al*. (1979) Patient Perceptions and Compliance. Recent studies of the health belief model. In: *Compliance in health care*. Johns Hopkins University Press, Baltimore.

Greenfield S and Kaplan SH *et al*. (1988) Patient's participation in medical care. *J Gen Intern Med*. **88:** 448-57.

Hays R (1990) Measuring consultation process. *PEGP*. **1:** 139-47.

Martin E *et al*. (1991) Why patients consult and what happens when they do. *BMJ*. **303:** 289-92.

Osmond H (1980) God and the doctor. *NEJM*. **302:** 555-8.

Savage R and Armstrong D (1990) The effect of a GP's consulting style on patients' satisfaction: a controlled study. *BMJ*. **301:** 968-70.

Stott NCH and Davis RH (1979) The exceptional potential in each primary care consultation. *JRCGP*. **29:** 201-5.

Waitzkin H and Stoeckle JD (1972) The communication of information about illness. *Adv Psychosom Med*. **8:** 180-215.

Wilson A (1991) Consultation length in general practice: a review. *BJGP*. **41:** 119-22.

Index